OBESITY

Selected Titles in ABC-CLIO's
CONTEMPORARY
WORLD ISSUES
Series

For a complete list of titles in this series, please visit
www.abc-clio.com.

Books in the Contemporary World Issues series address vital issues in today's society, such as genetic engineering, pollution, and biodiversity. Written by professional writers, scholars, and nonacademic experts, these books are authoritative, clearly written, up-to-date, and objective. They provide a good starting point for research by high school and college students, scholars, and general readers as well as by legislators, businesspeople, activists, and others.

Each book, carefully organized and easy to use, contains an overview of the subject, a detailed chronology, biographical sketches, facts and data and/or documents and other primary-source material, a directory of organizations and agencies, annotated lists of print and nonprint resources, and an index.

Readers of books in the Contemporary World Issues series will find the information they need to have a better understanding of the social, political, environmental, and economic issues facing the world today.

OBESITY

A Reference Handbook

Judith S. Stern and Alexandra Kazaks

**CONTEMPORARY
WORLD ISSUES**

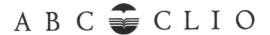

A B C 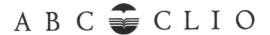 C L I O

Santa Barbara, California
Denver, Colorado
Oxford, England

Library of Congress Cataloging-in-Publication Data

Stern, Judith S., 1943–
  Obesity : a reference handbook / Judith Stern and
  Alexandra Kazaks.
    p. ; cm. — (Contemporary world issues)
  Includes bibliographical references and index.
  ISBN 978-1-59884-195-4 (hardcover : alk. paper)
  1. Obesity—Handbooks, manuals, etc. I. Kazaks, Alexandra. II. Title.
III. Series: Contemporary world issues.   [DNLM: 1. Obesity—United
States—Handbooks. WD 200.1 S839o 2009]
RA645.O23S74   2009
616.3'98—dc22   2009008131

13 12 11 10 9   1 2 3 4 5

E-ISBN: 978-1-59884-196-1

This book is also available on the World Wide Web as an eBook.

Visit www.abc-clio.com for details.

ABC-CLIO, LLC
130 Cremona Drive, P.O. Box 1911
Santa Barbara, California 93116-1911

This book is printed on acid-free paper ∞

Manufactured in the United States of America

Contents

List of Tables

List of Figures

Preface

We are obesity researchers and nutritionists. When people find out what we do, we are bombarded with questions like, Why are Americans so fat? How much should I weigh? What do you think about this diet? Is obesity such a problem in other countries? In order to answer these questions, we have written this reference book about obesity. We call it *Obesity* because factors like serving or being served very large portions, eating lots of fast food, and watching many hours of TV each day are significant problems in the United States.

This volume examines why people gain weight, why they either succeed or fail in losing it, and who they believe bears responsibility. You will learn about obesity treatments, important people in the obesity story, a wide range of resources, and interesting Web sites to keep you up-to-date. Included are discussions of controversial topics such as whether obesity is actually a disease. Chapter 1 defines obesity and its measures and gives a historical perspective. For example, obesity can be traced back to the Stone Age, and, historically, it was the wealthy who were obese. In fact, the famous 17th-century artist Peter Paul Rubens painted women who were "ideals of female beauty" who today would be considered obese. Furthermore, Chapter 1 explores how we have come to determine whether a person is at the "correct" weight

Chapter 2 discusses key problems, solutions, and controversies. For instance, are we really in the midst of an obesity epidemic? Is obesity a disease or a moral failing? Presented in this chapter is a section on how to make individualized plans, which includes how to assess your diet, reduce energy intake, and recognize fat as a concentrated source of energy. Some of the behavioral strategies demonstrate how to maintain a healthy weight while living in an obesogenic environment. The section on herbs and supplements identifies advertising claims that are, in fact, too good to be true. The pros and cons of various types of obesity surgery are discussed, and a provocative discussion is included of how the health care system deals with obesity. This chapter concludes with the thought that our biology, the influences of food advertising, and the customs of social eating act together to make obesity hard to prevent and treat.

Chapter 3 describes how overweight and obesity are dramatically increasing, not only in the United States but also in developing nations. The number of children who are overweight or obese has increased throughout the world. The highest rates of obesity are in the South Pacific; 70 percent of people living on the island of Nauru are now obese, whereas in the 1960s, only 15 percent were obese. The World Health Organization classifies obesity as one of the top risks to human health.

Chapter 4 presents a timeline of key discoveries, thinkers, and practices from 1942 to 2008.

Chapter 5 provides more than 50 short biographies of people who have been important in studying, preventing, managing, and increasing awareness about obesity. It includes people like Jared Fogle, who lost almost 245 pounds eating sandwiches from Subway; Ray Kroc, who started McDonald's fast food restaurants; Kelly Brownell, who coined the phrase "toxic environment" to describe our food and exercise patterns that contribute to obesity; and researcher Ethan Allen Sims, who coined the word "diabesity" to explain the relationship between obesity and diabetes. Oprah Winfrey, who said that if there was a pill to lose weight or a magic diet, she would have it, is also profiled.

Chapter 6 includes excerpts of key documents from the National Institutes of Health; the U.S. Surgeon General; and the National Heart, Lung and Blood Institute that guide how we view, prevent, and treat obesity. Also provided in this chapter are surprising facts as well as graphic figures and tables that depict some of the points made in chapters 1, 2, and 3.

Chapter 7 lists a variety of government, international, nonprofit, and trade and professional organizations and their Web sites. Some organizations promote health, study diseases, and provide statistics about health. Others, including the American Academy of Pediatrics, make available guides to childhood and adult obesity.

Chapter 8 lists a number of resources for additional in-depth information. Many are Web sites for government agencies such as the U.S. Department of Agriculture (www.usda.gov), Centers for Disease Control and Prevention (www.cdc.gov), and the National Institutes of Health (www.nih.gov). These sites provide reliable statistics and information about the latest research. Videos, such as *Super Size Me*, and books are listed that provide more background on the topic.

We really enjoyed writing this book and hope that you will use it as *the* reference book for obesity in the United States. We want to give special thanks to Brittany Smolen for her research.

1

Background and History

Obesity is not a recent phenomenon. Its origins can be traced back to our prehistoric ancestors. Statues dating from the Stone Age provide the earliest depiction of obesity. The Venus of Willendorf is a figurine of an obese woman that dates back to about 22,000 BCE. It is thought to represent a fertility goddess. Through the centuries obesity has been depicted in the arts, literature, and medical opinion both as a highly desirable state and as an unhealthy condition to be avoided. Egyptian temples prominently displayed statues of obese men and women while medical opinions written on papyrus at the time describe obesity as a disease state. Hippocrates, known as the father of medicine, noted that fat people were more prone to sudden death than were lean people. Stories and chronicles from the Middle Ages portray obese individuals who are wealthy and powerful. Peter Paul Rubens, a well-respected artist of the 17th century, painted ample, robust women who today would be labeled as obese but were considered ideals of female beauty at that time. In 1737 Benjamin Franklin observed in his Poor Richard's *Almanack*: "To lengthen thy life, lessen thy meals" (Franklin 1737). In the 1930s, it was rumored that the Duchess of Windsor declared, "You can never be too rich or too thin," setting a benchmark for socialites then and now.

Although overweight was sometimes linked with disease and a shorter life span, in general, extra fat was related to wealth, health, and attractiveness. Low weight and thinness were associated with poverty, malnutrition, and wasting diseases such as tuberculosis. Scarcity of food throughout most of history meant that most people did not have the opportunity to become obese. The tendency to store energy in the form of fat results from thousands of years of evolution in an environment characterized by limited or uncertain food supplies. Those who could store energy in times of plenty were more likely to survive periods of famine and to pass this tendency to their offspring. Obesity as a disease with pathologic consequences for a large percentage of the general public is less than a century old. The current availability of inexpensive, high-energy food and the reduced need to expend energy for daily living and work has allowed obesity to become an "equal opportunity" state of health.

Attitudes about body weight have fluctuated with the times. In the mid-19th century, the health reformer Sylvester Graham declared that overeating, or gluttony, was a great threat to both health and morality in the United States. In Graham's view, gluttony led to a state of what he called "over stimulation" that would eventually lead to illness and moral failings (Luciano 2001). During America's Gilded Age (1878–1889), fat bodies were equated with fat wallets, while thinness was associated with poverty. Rich men were depicted in the media with gold watch chains stretched across their ample bellies. The fashion of overindulgence was embodied by Diamond Jim Brady, a railroad equipment salesman who was known for his voracious appetite. A typical meal for Brady could include three dozen oysters, six crabs, soup, a half-dozen lobsters, two ducks, steak, vegetables, and a platter of desserts, followed by a two-pound box of candy. When he died at age 56, an autopsy showed his stomach was six times the size of that of a normal man. The fat person as a positive model did not persist past the 19th century. President William Taft, who weighed 355 pounds when he took office and suffered the indignity of getting stuck in the White House bathtub, was the last obese president (Luciano 2001).

A number of reasons explain this turnaround in attitudes about fatness. In the early 1920s, movies began to play a major role in shaping ideals of bodily perfection. Movie stars radiated youth, good health, and sex appeal. To look beautiful on film, actors and actresses had to be slim because filming on camera created the illusion that they carried extra pounds. From 1930 into the 1950s, it became fashionable for women to have a fuller bust and slender waist. Women were wearing girdles to narrow their waists and padded bras to enhance their breast line. Following World War II, fuller shapes became the accepted norm for housewives and mothers. Actresses like Jayne Mansfield and Marilyn Monroe, with their hourglass figures, were the voluptuous female ideal. During the late 1960s and early 1970s, the feminist movement questioned existing female stereotypes. The self-health movement at the time encouraged women to take pride in their body. This new concern of women about health and fitness fostered an industry that promoted cellulite creams, exercises to develop so-called buns of steel, and liposuction to remove unwanted fat. After the 1970s, a new, more athletic look became popular as increasing numbers of men and women began to participate in sports and regular exercise. In spite of the continuing popularity of the athletic body type, the prevailing look among top fashion models has remained ultrathin.

Through television, movies, and magazines, the media set unrealistic standards for desirable body weight and appearance. And portrayal of what is attractive and healthy keeps getting thinner and thinner for women and more muscular for men. At the beginning of the 21st century, two-thirds of Americans were overweight. In the next decades the population is expected to include a greater proportion of older people. The media image of health and beauty will be increasingly out of step with a population that is growing older and fatter.

The belief that weight and health could—and should—be under one's personal control generated a proliferation of dieting plans and treatments. One of the first commercially available diets came from William Banting in 1864. It was based on a high-protein and high-fat "low farinaceous" plan recommended to him by his doctor. Enthusiastic about his weight loss, he published the diet as "A Letter on Corpulence, Addressed to the Public" (Banting 1864). The plan became so popular that people spoke of "banting" when they went on any weight loss diet. Before the pure food and drug laws were passed in the United States, individuals seeking a cure-all for obesity were treated with doses of such products as vinegar and soap. Other ingredients used extensively in the 1920s that produced almost instant weight reduction were laxatives, which caused diarrhea, and purgatives, which induced vomiting. In the early 1900s, popular weight-loss drugs included a wide array of animal-derived thyroid, arsenic, and strychnine. Each could cause temporary weight loss, but they were unsafe to use. Newspapers of the time carried advertisements for Kellogg's Safe Fat Reducer, a much-promoted remedy that contained an extract of animal thyroid glands. Through a combination of aggressive advertising and questionable ethics, Kellogg's became a popular remedy for people seeking rapid weight loss. It was eventually revealed that the Safe Fat Reducer was a combination of thyroid extract, some laxatives, and bread-crumbs. Thyroid hormone as the active ingredient increased risk of hypertension, cardiac arrest, and stroke. Long-term use could result in loss of normal thyroid function, osteoporosis, increased heart rate, sweating, chest pain, and sudden death. The American Medical Association was successful in getting the thyroid extract removed from the product. However, it remained on the market and sold simply as a laxative.

For decades thyroid hormone was medically prescribed for obesity with the hope that an increase in metabolic rate would result in weight loss. Long-term studies demonstrated that weight loss occurring during thyroid hormone administration was due in part to the breakdown of vital protein as well as unwanted fat. In the 1930s, doctors prescribed dinitrophenol, a benzene-derived ingredient in World War I explosives. Dinitrophenol did increase metabolism and produced weight loss, but the drug was aban-doned because of severe side effects, including neuropathy and cataracts. During that time it was legal to sell untested remedies because drugmakers were not required to prove that their prod-ucts were safe before they were put on the market.

Defining and Measuring Overweight and Obesity

Defining overweight and obesity is somewhat subjective and imprecise. "Overweight" is defined as having more body weight than is considered normal or healthy for one's age or build. The term "obese" is used for very overweight people who have a high percentage of body fat. Normal weights have been vari-ously referred to as "ideal," "desirable," or "healthy." In addi-tion to these subjective terms are several objective measures that are used to classify individual weight.

Indirect Measuring Methods
Height-Weight Tables
In 1942, Louis Dublin, a statistician at Metropolitan Life Insur-ance Company, grouped some 4 million people who were insured with Metropolitan Life into categories based on their

height, body frame (small, medium, or large), and weight. He discovered that those who lived the longest were the people who maintained their body weight at the level for average 25-year-olds. The results were published in the Met Life standard height-weight tables for men and women, which were transformed from a record of national averages of weight in relation to age, sex, and height to the accepted guides for a healthy weight (MLIC 1942, 1943). The "1942–1943 Metropolitan Height and Weight Tables" shown in Table 6.1 in Chapter 6 became widely used for determining "ideal" body weights.

In 1959, research indicated that the lowest mortality rates were associated with lower-than-average weights, and the phrase "desirable weight" replaced "ideal weight" in the height and weight table (MLIC 1959). The weights were derived from those weight-for-height proportions associated with lowest mortality among people in the United States and Canada who purchased life insurance policies from 1935 to 1954. However, these weights were associated with the lowest death rates but not necessarily with the lowest morbidity (rate of illness or disease). In 1983, the tables were revised once again and called simply "height and weight tables." The weights given in the 1983 tables are heavier than the 1942 tables because, in general, heavier people were living longer (MLIC 1983). It is interesting to note that neither medical nor academic experts were the authoritative voices in setting weight guidelines. It was the life insurance industry that established the system of weight classification that became part of medical practice throughout the United States.

A number of criticisms surrounded the use of a table to determine whether an individual is at the right weight—or even what "ideal weight" means. Experts have criticized the validity of the Met Life tables for several reasons:

- Insured people tend to be healthier than uninsured people.
- Frame size was not consistently measured.
- The tables were based on a predominantly white, middle-class population.
- Some individuals were actually weighed and some reported their estimated weight.
- Height and weight were measured in people wearing shoes and clothing of varying amounts and weights.

- Both smokers and nonsmokers were included. Smoking is a significant factor that increases risk of disease and death.

Thus, height-weight tables should be used only as a guide, and other measurements should be included for health evaluation.

People in the United States were able to find out how much they weighed when penny scales were imported from Germany in the 1880s. Soon after, the National Scale Company manufactured the first coin-operated scales in the United States. These scales were among the first automatic vending machines. Being able to weigh oneself was a novelty at the time, and during the 1920s and 1930s, coin-operated scales appeared in drugstores in almost every city and town. In the 1940s, improvements in mechanical scale technology made inexpensive personal scales available for in-home use. Today, we can choose bathroom scales that are digital, that are solar powered, or that "talk" and say the weight aloud. The accuracy in these scales may vary, but they serve the general purpose of measuring whether body weight is going up or down.

Estimated Ideal Body Weight

In 1964, Dr. G. J. Hamwi developed a simple rule for estimating ideal body weight (IBW). The Hamwi formulas have become very popular since they first appeared in a publication of the American Diabetes Association (Hamwi 1964). They have remained a well-accepted method of calculating ideal weight in clinical situations. The formulas for IBW are:

Men—106 pounds for the first 5 feet; 6 pounds for each inch over 5 feet

Women—100 pounds for the first 5 feet; 5 pounds for each inch over 5 feet

In addition, a range of 10 percent variation above or below the calculated weight was allowed for individual differences.

Example:

The estimated ideal body weight of a man who is 5 feet, 11 inches tall would be calculated as:

$$106 + (6 \times 11) = 106 + 66 = \textbf{172 pounds}$$

The range with 10 percent variation below and above is **155 to 189 pounds** (10 percent of 172 = about 17 pounds, so 172 − 17 = 155 and 172 + 17 = 189).

The estimated ideal body weight of a woman who is 5 feet 4 inches tall would be calculated as:

$$100 + (5 \times 4) = 100 + 20 = \textbf{120 pounds}$$

The range with 10 percent variation below and above is **113 to 137 pounds** (10 percent of 120 = 12 pounds, so 125 − 12 = 113 and 125 + 12 = 137).

The IBW does not correlate weight to health or prevention of disease. One criticism of the IBW formula is that it does not allow for body composition or body type. Someone with large bones or with a high percentage of lean tissue (muscle) would appear to be overweight according to this method. For some, the IBW may be an unrealistic range, and they may try unnecessary or fad dieting to reach the "ideal" number.

Body Mass Index

As definitions of overweight have varied widely, health experts have struggled to develop a useful definition of healthy weight. Their recommendations have evolved from weight-for-height standards to sex-specific references. The most recent proposal is to use a single number, the body mass index (BMI) that is applied to all adults. BMI is a calculated number, based on height and weight of an individual. It is calculated as:

$$\textbf{BMI = weight (lb)/[height (in)]}^2 \times \textbf{703}$$
(standard units of measure)

or as:

$$\textbf{BMI = weight (kg)/[height (m)]}^2 \text{ (metric units of measure)}$$

where kg = kilogram, m = meter, lb = pound, and in = inch.

This number is used to analyze health effects of body weight. Because it is independent of age and reference population, BMI can be used for comparisons across studies both in the United States and internationally. The BMI is more generous than the IBW. BMI calculations are meant to be applied only to adults over age 20. At age two, children can be given a BMI number; however, they are rated differently from adults.

BMI can be calculated in inches and pounds (in the United States) or in meters and kilograms (in countries that use the metric system).

One can calculate BMI by dividing weight in pounds by height in inches squared and multiplying that number by a conversion factor of 703.

Example:

If one's weight is 150 pounds and height is 5′5″ (65″), the BMI is calculated as:

$$[150 \div (65)^2] \times 703 = 24.96$$

With the metric system, the formula for BMI is weight in kilograms divided by height in meters squared.

Example:

If one's weight is 68 kilograms and height is 165 centimeters (1.65 meters), the BMI is calculated as:

$$68 \div (1.65)^2 = 24.98$$

One can use available tables to easily determine BMI (see Table 6.2 in Chapter 6) or enter one's weight and height into a Web-based BMI calculator. One such calculator is made available by the Centers for Disease Control and Prevention (CDC) at http://www.cdc.gov/nccdphp/dnpa/bmi/.

Based upon guidelines from the National Heart, Lung and Blood Institute and the World Health Organization, Table 1.1 shows weight ranges compared with BMI values used to determine weight status.

TABLE 1.1
Weight Ranges, BMI Values, and Weight Status

Height	Weight Range	BMI	Considered
5′ 9″	124 lb. or less	Below 18.5	Underweight
	125 lb. to 168 lb.	18.5 to 24.9	Healthy weight
	169 lb. to 202 lb.	25.0 to 29.9	Overweight
	203 lb. or more	30 or higher	Obese

Note: This example is for a person 5 feet 9 inches tall.

Source: CDC (2007a).

The BMI was first developed in the mid-1800s by a Belgian mathematician named Adolphe Quetelet. Quetelet worked with life insurance companies to determine factors related to birth and death. These types of correlations using body weight are common now, but in 1833 the idea was revolutionary. More recently, governmental agencies and scientific health organizations have defined a BMI that correlates with the health risks of overweight using a statistically derived definition from a series of cross-sectional surveys called the National Health and Nutrition Examination Surveys (NHANES). These surveys are designed to gather information on the health and nutritional status of the population of the United States. From 1985 to 1998, the definition of overweight in government publications was a BMI of at least 27.3 for women and 27.8 for men.

In 1995, the World Health Organization recommended a new classification system that included three "grades" of overweight using BMI cutoff points of 25, 30, and 40. The International Obesity Task Force suggested an additional cutoff point of 35. Eventually, in June 1998, an expert panel convened by the National Institutes of Health (NIH) released a report that identified being overweight as having a BMI between 25 and 29.9 and being obese as having a BMI of 30 or above. These definitions, widely used by the federal government and increasingly used by the broader medical and scientific communities, are based on evidence that health risks increase more steeply in individuals with a BMI greater than 25. The term "morbid obesity" is still used for medical coding purposes for individuals with a BMI of 40 or above; however, the NIH recommends the use of other descriptive terms, such as "Class III obesity," "extreme obesity," or "clinically severe obesity."

Use of BMI cutoffs has been varied, yielding contrasting results. A shift in BMI criteria can have a large effect on the population at risk (Kuczmarski and Flegal 2000). For example, when applying the BMI cutoffs of ≥27.8 for men and ≥27.3 for women to NHANES III—data collected between 1988 and 1994—the prevalence of overweight is 33 percent for men and 36 percent for women (CDC 1999). In contrast, with the lower BMI cutoff of ≥25.0, the prevalence is 59 percent among men and 51 percent among women. Changing the overweight group cutoff increases the estimated number of overweight adults from 61.7 million to 97.1 million, putting 35.4 million more adults into the overweight category.

Limitations and Shortcomings

Measuring body weight and body dimensions—or anthropometry—is a quick and inexpensive way to estimate body fatness. However, using calculated numbers such as BMI does have limitations. A problem with using BMI as a measurement tool is that very muscular people may be classified as overweight when they are actually healthy. Similarly, people who have lost muscle mass, such as the elderly, may have a weight that is in the healthy BMI category when they actually have a high percentage of body fat. The health risks associated with overweight and obesity are based on a continuum and do not necessarily correspond to strict cutoff points. For example, an overweight individual with a BMI of 29 does not substantially add to his or her health consequences simply by moving up one notch to a BMI of 30, the threshold of the obese category (WIN 2006). Because health risks generally do increase with increasing BMI, it is a useful screening tool for individuals and a general guideline to monitor trends in the population. By itself, BMI is not diagnostic for individual health status. Further assessment should be performed to evaluate associated health risks.

BMI ranges for children and teens are defined so that they take into account normal differences between boys and girls at various ages. After BMI is calculated, the BMI number is plotted on BMI-for-age growth charts specific for either girls or boys to obtain a percentile ranking. The percentile indicates the relative position of the child's BMI number among children of the same sex and age. The Centers for Disease Control and Prevention BMI-for-age weight status categories and the corresponding percentiles are shown in Table 1.2.

The CDC provides more information about BMI for children and teens at an interactive Web site, http://www.cdc.gov/nccdphp/dnpa/healthyweight/assessing/bmi/childrens_BMI/about_childrens_BMI.htm.

Debate is ongoing among researchers and health professionals about whether BMI is a reasonable indicator of body fatness, as the correlation between the BMI and body fatness can vary greatly according to sex, age, and race. For example:

- At the same BMI, women tend to have more body fat than men.

TABLE 1.2
Children's BMI-for-Age Weight Status

Weight Status Category	Percentile Range (compared with boys or girls of same age)
Underweight	Less than the 5th percentile
Healthy weight	5th percentile to less than the 85th percentile
At risk of overweight	85th to less than the 95th percentile
Overweight	Equal to or greater than the 95th percentile

Source: CDC (2007a).

- At the same BMI, older people, on average, tend to have more body fat than younger adults.
- Race and ethnicity issues are inherent in BMI measurements.

BMI does not take into account how people of different races and ethnicities vary in muscle mass versus fat mass. People of African and Polynesian ancestry may have less body fat and more lean muscle mass for a given weight, and thus a higher baseline BMI for overweight and obesity may be appropriate for these populations. At the other end of the scale, one study found that current BMI thresholds significantly underestimate health risks in many non-Europeans (Gallagher 2004). The body fat percentage of an Asian would be higher than that of a Caucasian of the same height and weight. Even within normal BMI ranges, Asian groups have a high risk of weight-related health problems, and they begin to have abnormalities in their blood glucose levels above a BMI of 21. It has been suggested that BMI levels be dropped to 23 and 25 for overweight and obesity, respectively, among Asian populations (Razak et al. 2007).

Assessing Percentage of Body Fat

BMI is not a specific index of fatness because its numerator—measured body weight—may reflect muscle, bone, or body water in addition to fat. The percentage of body fat is difficult to measure directly. Fat, or adipose, tissue is stored underneath the skin as subcutaneous fat; as intramuscular fat, interspersed in skeletal muscle; and as visceral adipose tissue, found deep in the body around vital organs. Body fat can be divided into two categories according to its physiological purpose: Essential fat cushions and insulates organs and is necessary for normal body function. Nonessential fat is excess energy stored away for future use. Although no universal body fat standards are in place, the American Council on Exercise has suggested an average amount of body fat of 18 to 24 percent for men and 25 to 31 percent for women. Any amount over that range would be considered obesity (ACSM 2001).

The distribution of adipose tissue is important, because overweight and obese adults are divided into risk categories depending on body shape and location of fat deposits. "Pear shaped" individuals, who have fat deposits on their hips and thighs, are less susceptible to obesity-related diseases than "apple shaped" people, who store fat in the abdominal area. Abdominal fat accumulation is generally considered to be a key health risk indicator, as increased waist circumference is associated strongly with cardiovascular disease and is a good predictor of future risk of type 2 diabetes and all-cause mortality. Measuring waist circumference is a simple procedure that provides information about fat distribution, but it is unclear how commonly clinicians measure waist circumference. Anecdotal evidence suggests that this practice is not routine. As part of a complete health risk assessment, health care professionals are urged to incorporate waist circumference along with measuring weight, height, and BMI calculations (Ford, Mokdad, and Giles 2003).

Direct Measuring Methods

Direct measures of body fat include underwater weighing, bioelectrical impedance analysis (BIA), dual energy X-ray absorptiometry (DEXA), and skinfold thickness. These measures of body fat can be expensive or time consuming and are not normally used by primary care clinicians. However, they can complement BMI to assess risk and monitor the progress of therapeutic interventions (Erselcan et al. 2000).

Underwater Weighing

Underwater weighing, also known as densitometry or hydrostatic weighing, has long been the gold standard for determining body composition (relative amounts of fat and lean). This technique involves weighing a person when dry and then measuring his or her weight when totally submerged in a tub of water and the air in the lungs has been fully exhaled. It is based on Archimedes' principle, which states that given an equal weight, lower-density objects have a larger surface area and displace more water than higher-density objects. Bone and muscle are denser than water and sinks, and fat is less dense than water and floats. Of two individuals of the same weight but with different proportions of fat and lean, the one with the most body fat weighs less under water. The volume of water displaced by a person and the difference between the dry weight and the submerged weight are entered into equations that can be used to estimate percentage of body fat. The primary disadvantages of this method are the cost and time required, the subject having to be underwater, and the variability in the ability of individuals to fully exhale. This technique is not a useful approach for large-scale studies, and in terms of precision, a DEXA scan is an alternative.

Dual Energy X-ray Absorptiometry

With DEXA, a scanner measures body composition using low energy X-rays. This method was originally developed to evaluate changes in bone mineral density, but it also reveals total body composition. DEXA works by passing two X-ray beams through the individual and measuring the amount of X-ray absorbed by the tissue it has passed through. One beam is high intensity and one is low intensity, so the relative absorbance of each beam is an indication of the density of the tissue. DEXA differentiates fat from lean mass, as tissue with greater density (e.g., bone and muscle) shows a greater reduction in X-ray that passes through and that can be detected. The amount of radiation energy that is used with DEXA is extremely small. It would take approximately 800 full-body DEXA scans to equal the exposure to the amount of radiation received from one standard chest X-ray. The level of radiation is low enough that DEXA is approved by the U.S. Food and Drug Administration as a screening device to predict body composition. DEXA is a very accurate measure of body fat, although it is expensive and is generally limited to clinical research studies (Bolanowski and Nilsson 2001).

Bioelectrical Impedance Analysis

BIA is based on the principle that body tissue is capable of conducting electricity. Water is a good conductor of electricity, and most body water is found in lean tissue. Fat, which has almost no water in it, is such a poor conductor of electricity that it actually impedes, or slows down, the electrical flow. High measured resistance equals a high level of fat. Impedance is calculated by entering the resistance data into regression equations that take into account the person's weight, age, gender, and ethnicity. The BIA method is population specific, and an equation must be used that is specific to the population being measured (Heymsfield et al. 1996). Although this type of measurement initially required a laboratory procedure that involved attaching electrodes to the hands and feet, the technology now features easy-to-use devices, including at-home floor scales. BIA is considered to be safe because BIA currents (at a frequency of 50 kilohertz) are unlikely to stimulate electrically excitable tissues, such as nerves or cardiac muscle. The small current magnitudes are less than the threshold of perception—that is, they are not noticeable. Anyone with an implanted defibrillator should avoid BIA evaluation because even small currents could potentially provoke an incorrect defibrillator response (NHLBI 1998).

Measurement

Skinfold measurement is an inexpensive option for estimating body fat based on the assumption that subcutaneous fat reflects the total fat content of the body. Calipers are used to measure subcutaneous fat at specific sites around the body, including the chest, hip, abdomen, thigh, and upper arm. Prediction equations that help estimate body fat from skinfold sites can be examined in Table 6.3 in Chapter 6.

The skinfold technique is prone to significant measurement errors. Limitations on how wide the calipers open can make skinfold measurement challenging to use with extremely obese patients. In addition, not all body fat, such as intra-abdominal and intramuscular fat, is accessible to the calipers, and the distribution of subcutaneous fat can vary significantly throughout the human body. Although skinfold measurements are easily administered and are practical for large studies, they have been found to provide the least accurate estimates of percentage of body fat (Wang et al. 2000).

Obesity Trends in the United States

According to the National Center for Health Statistics (NCHS), an agency connected with the CDC, 66 percent of U.S. adults

TABLE 1.3
Prevalence of Overweight and Obesity among U.S. Adults, Age 20 Years and Over (%)

	NHANES III (1988–94)	NHANES (1999–2000)	NHANES (2001–02)	NHANES (2003–04)
Percent overweight or obese (BMI greater than or equal to 25.0)	56.0	64.5	65.7	66.3
Percent obese (BMI greater than or equal to 30.0)	22.9	30.5	30.6	32.2

Source: CDC (2007b).

age 20 years and older are either overweight or obese (NCHS 2006). The NCHS has been gathering data about obesity in the United States since 1960. In the first survey, almost 13 percent of the population was obese. Obesity rates showed a slight increase up to 1976–1980, then a rapid rise. More than twice as many U.S. men and women were classified as obese in 1999–2000 as in 1960. Table 1.3 illustrates how obesity has increased in American adults to the point that 3 out of 10 are obese.

The continuing trend of increasing obesity in the United States can be seen in Figure 6.1 in Chapter 6, "Obesity Trends Among U.S. Adults," showing the prevalence of obesity across each state. This increase in prevalence has occurred among all racial and ethnic groups; in men, women, and children; among all educational levels; and throughout all regions of the United States. However, some groups have consistently seen higher prevalence than others. In 2006, the southeastern region of the United States had the highest prevalence of obesity and overweight, led by Mississippi and West Virginia, which each had a prevalence of obesity equal to or greater than 30 percent of its population.

Since 1980, a similar increase in overweight has been seen among children and adolescents. Table 1.4 shows NHANES 1999–2004 estimates of overweight among young people compared with prior and later NHANES figures. The data suggest that overweight in this population has been consistently increasing since it was first measured in 1963.

Although there is no generally accepted definition for "obesity" as distinct from "overweight" in children and adolescents, NCHS data show that between the 1976–1980 and 2003–2004 surveys, the prevalence of overweight was as follows:

TABLE 1.4
Prevalence of Overweight among Children and Adolescents

Age (years)	NHANES 1963–65, 1966–70	NHANES 1971–74	NHANES 1988–94	NHANES 1999–2000	NHANES 2001–02	NHANES 2003–04
6–11	4.2	4.0	11.3	15.1	16.3	18.8
12–19	4.6	6.1	10.5	14.8	16.7	17.4

Source: NCHS (2006).

- Increased from 5.0 percent to 13.9 percent among preschool-age children, age 2–5 years.
- Increased from 4.0 percent to 18.8 percent among school-age children, age 6–11 years.
- Increased from 6.1 percent to 17.4 percent among school-age adolescents, age 12–19 years (NCHS 2006).

A young person with excess weight has a high risk of obesity-related health problems in the future. Overweight adolescents have a 70 percent chance of becoming overweight or obese adults. Heart disease related to high cholesterol and high blood pressure occurs with increased frequency in overweight young people compared with those with a healthy weight. Type 2 diabetes, closely linked to overweight and obesity and previously considered an adult disease, has increased significantly in children and adolescents. Experts harbor serious concerns that the current generation of children will experience debilitating chronic diseases in adulthood and will actually have a shorter life span than their parents (Olshansky et al. 2005).

Obesity as a National Health Problem

When Brandreth Symonds, a life insurance statistician, published "The Influence of Overweight and Underweight on Vitality" in 1908, his statistical analysis of insurance policyholders showed that overweight was a greater risk factor for a shortened life span than underweight. Dr. Symonds wrote, "Speaking generally, it is safer to be thin than fat" (Symonds 1908).

In 1943, enough of the U.S. population was above the IBW that the Metropolitan Life Insurance Company declared, "Overweight is so common that it constitutes a national health problem of the first order" (MLIC 1943). In a classic paper, Dr. Lester Breslow noted that "one out of six 'well people' . . . were 20 percent or more overweight" and that weight control was a "major public health problem" (Breslow 1952). The obesity prevalence estimates in Breslow's paper are small compared with current figures showing that 65 percent of U.S. adults are now classified as overweight or obese. Former U.S. Surgeon General David Satcher declared obesity to be a "public health epidemic" in the 2001 publication "Surgeon General's Call to Action to Prevent and Decrease Overweight and Obesity." He said, "Health problems resulting from overweight and obesity could reverse many of the health gains achieved in the U.S. in recent decades" (HHS 2001).

Healthy People 2010, a U.S. Department of Health and Human Services health promotion and disease prevention program, highlights overweight and obesity as key indicators of national health. It set an objective to reduce the prevalence of obesity among adults to less than 15 percent. The United States has made little progress toward that target. In fact, current data indicate that the obesity situation is getting worse.

Why Are We Overweight?

The obesity crisis did not happen overnight. It has been developing for decades, but only recently has it attracted much public attention. The U.S. population has experienced steady gains in both weight and height since the late 19th century. These gains improved our capability to withstand diseases and increased our longevity. Between 1900 and 2000, life expectancy at birth in the United States increased by 65 percent for women and by 60 percent for men. Gains in height among U.S. adults have leveled off, and weight has continued to increase. As obesity and overweight have risen in our population, the greatest increase in the past two decades has been seen in the prevalence of extreme obesity. Those who are severely obese are most at risk for serious health problems (NHLBI 1998; NIH 1998).

Most people are aware of the health problems associated with excess weight. Diet books top the best-seller list and the electronic and print media are loaded with nutrition advice, but successful individual weight management is haphazard or even nonexistent. Why are Americans overweight? Is it the availability of fast food? Oversized portions? Too much TV? Experts argue about the causes or contributors to overweight and obesity, but the realistic answer is, too many calories. The reality is that we eat too much and move too little. At the most fundamental level, weight gain is caused by the imbalance between food and activity: too much energy in and too little energy out. Weight gain is the normal physiologic response that occurs when energy intake exceeds energy expenditure.

Obesity is a consequence of our modern life. We have access to large amounts of palatable, high-calorie food and a limited need for physical activity. Humans evolved in an environment that required vigorous physical activity and was characterized by cyclical feast and famine. To survive, humans developed an innate preference for sweet and fatty foods. These natural defenses against starvation go awry in an environment where food is always plentiful and technology has reduced the need for human physical work. As the amount of energy, or calories, in our food supply has grown in recent decades, each person has consumed more food. Those extra calories turn into extra pounds year after year.

Food energy is measured in calories. A calorie is defined as the amount of energy (or heat) it takes to raise 1 gram of water (approximately 1 cubic centimeter, or about a thimbleful) 1°C. In nutrition terms, the word "calorie" is used instead of the more precise scientific term "kilocalorie," or 1,000 calories of energy. Dietary calories are in fact kilocalories (Kcal), with the "kilo-" prefix omitted. Here the terms are interchangeable, with Kcal used most often with numbers or measurements.

When extra energy in the form of protein (4 Kcal/gram), fat (9 Kcal/gram), carbohydrate (4 Kcal/gram) and/or alcohol (7 Kcal/gram) is consumed, the excess energy is stored in the form of body fat. Conversely, by limiting energy intake, body fat loss will be in proportion to the calorie deficit. Each pound of body fat represents approximately 3,500 Kcal. Reducing calorie intake by 500 Kcal per day theoretically results in a 1 pound per week weight loss. Small changes in food intake can make large differences over time. For example, using one tablespoon of mayonnaise on a sandwich instead of two tablespoons can save 100 calories per day. Over a year the total 36,500 Kcal (365 days ×

100 Kcal/day) deficit could mean a loss of 10 pounds of body fat. Most people have between 25 billion and 35 billion fat cells. This number can increase in response to excessive weight gain to as many as 150 billion cells. Fat cells expand and shrink in size during weight gain and loss, but they never disappear.

Because resting metabolic rate (the energy required to maintain basic physiologic functions and for digestion) varies widely among individuals, calorie intake and physical energy expenditure are the most variable components of energy balance. Changes in eating and activity provide the best opportunities to prevent or treat obesity (Goran 2000).

Despite concern about the increasing levels of obesity, and the knowledge that it is caused by excess energy intake and low levels of physical activity, obesity remains a poorly understood phenomenon. Considerable gaps remain in our knowledge about the physiological pathways underlying weight gain and the effectiveness of dietary, behavioral, and physical activity interventions. Americans, among the heaviest people on Earth, are becoming fatter and at an ever younger age. How we got to this point is an account of the complex interplay between biological, psychosocial, and economic factors.

Factors That Contribute to Obesity

To understand obesity, we must comprehend the dimensions of energy balance:

- Energy in: Factors that affect food consumption
- Energy out: Factors that affect activity level
- Metabolic and genetic contributions

Increased Energy Intake

The surge in obesity in the United States reflects an increase in per capita energy intake between 1970 and 1997 from 2,220 Kcal to 2,680 Kcal. These figures are estimated from the total food available in the national supply (Putnam, Kantor, and Allshouse 2000). Several factors have encouraged Americans to eat more. In the early 1980s, food production was an average of 3,300 calories a day for every person. Then U.S. farm policy changed, in a way that moved farmers toward lower price supports, greater planting flexibility and greater orientation to market forces. Farmers increased harvests and no longer plowed under food crops to get subsidies for reducing production. Today, American farmers produce enough food to allow every person 3,900 calories a day. Food prices in stores and restaurants have been declining relative to prices of all other items. Between 1952 and 2003, the ratio of food prices to the price of all other goods fell by 12 percent. Foods that once were available only seasonally are now available year-round, and advances in food processing and packaging have made available a multitude of ready-to-eat foods virtually anywhere at any time (Variyam 2005).

Preparing food is now also more convenient. In 1965, it took a housewife more than two hours per day to shop for, cook, and clean up from meals. By 1995, the time it took to do these tasks was cut in half. Researchers from Harvard University have suggested that the increase in food consumption permitted by the falling time cost of preparing and acquiring food is a major factor behind the surge in obesity since 1980 (Variyam 2005).

"A Nation at Risk: Obesity in the United States," published jointly by the American Heart Association and the Robert Wood Johnson Foundation in 2005, reported data from scientific research studies about changes in the eating patterns of Americans over the past few decades. Trends that contribute to obesity are:

1. More calories: Adults consumed approximately 300 more calories daily in 2000 than they did in 1985.
2. Bigger portion sizes: A study in the *Journal of the American Medical Association* cited in this study reported a significant rise in portion sizes from 1977 to 1996.
3. A major increase in eating out: Spending in fast-food restaurants grew 18 times (from $6 billion to $110 billion) in the past three decades. In 1970, approximately 30,000 fast-food restaurants were operating in the United States; in 2001, approximately 222,000 were in operation (AHA 2005).

Distorted Portion Sizes

Portion sizes have dramatically increased in the past 40 years. As we are exposed to larger quantities of food sold as a single portion, we become victims of "portion distortion." Many of the changes have been too subtle to notice; we have become used to larger servings, and we now expect them. Consider the maximum serving size of french fries sold at McDonald's. It has increased from 210 calories in 1955 to 610 calories. Greater increases are seen in the size of soft drinks. In the 1950s, the standard-size Coca Cola was about 6 ounces. At many U.S. convenience stores, 64-ounce (2 quarts) soft drinks are common.

The sizes of muffins, bagels, and croissants also contribute to portion distortion. Portion-size increases have been continuous since the 1970s. In a sample of 63,380 individuals who responded to national surveys conducted by the USDA between 1977 and 1998, food portion sizes consumed at home and in restaurants increased markedly (Nielsen and Popkin 2003):

- Salty snacks increased from 1.0 to 1.6 ounces = 93 more calories.
- Soft drinks increased from 13.1 to 19.9 fluid ounces = 49 more calories.
- Hamburgers increased from 5.7 to 7.0 ounces = 97 more calories.
- Mexican food increased from 6.3 to 8.0 ounces = 133 more calories.

Though it only costs a few cents more to get a larger size of french fries or a soft drink, the result is too many calories for one person. "Value meals" may not generate any savings when the monetary and psychological costs of trying to lose weight gained from eating larger portions are factored in. Large portion sizes are not limited to meals. Bags of snack foods or soft drinks in vending machines and grocery stores are available in larger and larger sizes that contain multiple servings. (The National Institutes of Health Web site, "Portion Distortion," has an interactive quiz to show how portions today compare with portion sizes 20 years ago. Visit http://hp2010.nhlbihin.net/portion/to view the quiz.)

What is the effect of larger portion sizes on food intake? According to research conducted by Professor Brian Wansink, people eat more if the product is being eaten from larger packages (Wansink and Kim 2005). He conducted a "popcorn test" demonstrating that people given large containers of popcorn ate an average of 44 percent more (equal to about 120 Kcal) than those who were given small containers, even though they said the popcorn did not taste very good. In a study by Rolls and colleagues, volunteers ate 30 percent more macaroni and cheese when given large 35 ounce portions than when they were given smaller 18 ounce portions during a meal (Rolls, Morris, and Roe 2002). Consumers eat more from large servings, but, more important, they also get a distorted impression of what a reasonable serving size really is.

Large food portions affect children's energy intake at meals, even among toddlers (Fisher et al. 2007). Children ranging in age from two to nine years were either given an age-appropriate entrée at the dinner meal or a portion size twice as large as the age-appropriate portion. The study results showed that children as young as two years had a 13 percent higher energy intake at the meal when given the large-portion entrée. Interestingly, children took a similar number of bites regardless of the portion size, but they took *bigger bites* when served the larger portion.

What Is the Difference between Portion Size and Serving Size?

Portion control is not easy. Standardized servings used to develop labeling laws and the U.S. Department of Agriculture Food Guide Pyramid are much smaller than portions commonly consumed. Portion size is the amount of a single food item served in a single eating occasion, such as a meal or a snack. A portion is the amount offered to a person in a restaurant, the amount offered in the packaging of prepared foods, or the quantity a person chooses to put on his or her plate.

Serving size is a standardized unit of measuring foods—for example, a cup or an ounce—used in the *Dietary Guidelines for Americans* and listed on a product label's nutrition facts. The portion and serving size may match, but frequently they are different. For example, bagels or muffins are often sold in portion sizes that comprise at least two servings. When consumers eat the whole product, they may think that they have eaten only a single serving (CDC 2006).

Food labels can help people understand that portions are often larger than they think. For example, one serving of potato or corn chips might supply just 100 calories. But when the serving size is only 10 chips and there are 10 servings per bag, the calories really add up if a person finishes the whole bag. The nutrition facts labels on beverage containers often give the calories for only part of the contents. The label on a 20-ounce bottle often lists the number of calories in an 8-ounce serving even though the bottle contains 20 ounces, or 2.5 servings. To figure out how many calories are in the whole bottle, one must multiply the number of calories in one serving by the number of servings in the bottle (100 × 2.5). The whole bottle actually contains 250 calories. It is important to look closely at the serving size when determining the calorie content of beverages. Note that the serving size on the nutrition facts label is not a recommended amount of food to eat; it is just the calories and nutrients in a given amount of food.

Drinking More Calories

Sugar-sweetened beverages, including sweetened fruit drinks and carbonated drinks, account for nearly half of the added sugars in the U.S. diet (Guthrie and Morton 2000). In 1997, 2.8 million vending machines dispensed more than 27 billion drinks. Most of those drinks came in 12-ounce cans, but the soft drink trend is toward serving sizes of 20 ounces or more. The larger the container, the more beverage people will drink, especially when they assume that the container is a single serving, whether it is 12 ounces, 20 ounces, or more (Johnson et al. 2007).

Soft drinks contribute extra energy that adds up day after day and eventually leads to overweight and obesity. Another reason to limit sugar-sweetened drinks is that liquid calories may not be recognized by the body's appetite feedback mechanisms. People normally adjust or moderate energy intake by eating less after a large meal, but that moderation occurs more readily with solid foods than with beverages. This phenomenon was seen in a study of men and women who were given 450 extra calories per day as either 3- to 12-ounce cans of soda or 45 large jelly beans. The people who ate the candy adjusted for the extra energy and later ate less. Those who got the extra liquid calories made no compensation afterward; subsequently, their overall calorie intake increased. The author of the article stated, "Liquid calories don't trip our satiety mechanisms. They just don't register" (DiMeglio and Mattes 2000).

Conveniently Available Food

Meals eaten away from home allow easy and often inexpensive access to large quantities of calorie-rich foods. In 1970, away-from-home meals represented 25 percent of households' total food budget. In 1995, that percentage had risen to 40 percent (Guthrie, Lin, and Frazao 2002). The National Restaurant Association reported that in 1981 the average American ate 3.7 commercially prepared meals per week. By 2000, that number had increased to 4.2 per week. All those meals have contributed to the increase in overweight and obesity, as the frequency of eating in restaurants has been positively associated with body fatness. Ample evidence exists to show that, ounce for ounce, foods eaten away from home are more calorie dense than foods prepared at home (McCrory et al. 1999). As the food service industry offers more choices, from fast food to a wide array of ethnic restaurants, the popularity of dining out implies that desire for convenience and variety overrides concern about obesity.

Physical Inactivity

Along with a growing tendency to consume more calories, Americans have become less active overall than they were 20 years ago. Given labor-saving devices, from personal automobiles to e-mail, and a technology-driven workforce that is shifting from physically demanding manual labor to sedentary work, we cannot expect daily caloric expenditure to increase. For most people daily work no longer provides the opportunity for physical activity that it once did. As jobs have become more sedentary, the workweek has been expanding, so even less time is available for leisure-time physical activity. Television viewing accounts for half of the average adult's leisure time in the United States (Hu et al. 2001).

The CDC and the Office of the Surgeon General recommend that all adults should do at least 30 minutes of moderate-intensity physical activity most days of the week. National statistics from 2000 indicate that only about 20 percent of Americans reached the minimum activity goal. This percentage of inactive people has not changed since the 1970s, but during that period the population increased by about 60 million people, meaning that the number of sedentary Americans actually increased by 48 million. Activity does not need to be high intensity or done all at one time to be beneficial. An example of a moderate-intensity activity is brisk walking (a pace of 15 to 20 minutes per mile) for 30 minutes. The 30 minutes can be divided into three walks of 10 minutes each and still meet the recommendation (CDC 2008).

Due to the reduction of physical education in schools, the lack of access to playgrounds, and concerns for physical safety, many children do not get the recommended amount of daily activity. Researchers at Johns Hopkins University reported that watching television is the number one leisure-time activity among school-age children. A study from 1998 indicated that more than a quarter of U.S. children watch four or more hours of television a day (Andersen et al. 1998). A more recent study reported that youth 6 to 13 years old spend approximately three hours per day watching television; however, when time spent on computers and video games is added, screen media exposure exceeds five hours per day (Jordan 2006). Television viewing affects childhood obesity in two ways: Watching TV is sedentary, and food consumption is increased when children eat while viewing programs or as they respond to the frequent advertisements of high-calorie fun and exciting foods by reaching for more snacks (Powell et al. 2007).

Physical Activity and Short-term Weight Loss

Physical activity has favorable effects on the body's metabolic systems, so numerous health benefits are gained from exercise even without weight loss. This point is important to keep in mind because, contrary to the belief that exercise causes weight loss, data from randomized controlled studies suggest that adding exercise to dietary therapy does not significantly increase short-term weight loss when compared with dieting without exercise (Wing 1999). Resistance exercise can build strength and muscle tissue, which may allow an obese or overweight person to become more physically active; however, neither resistance nor strength training increases weight loss (Jakicic et al. 2001, 2008). The ineffectiveness of moderate exercise alone to reduce body fat is not surprising when we consider that 1 pound of body fat contains the equivalent of about 3,500 Kcal, and to reduce body fat one must expend more energy than is taken in.

But moderate exercise is not useless. Depending on a person's body weight, 15 minutes of brisk walking uses about 100 Kcal. As shown in the list below, walking for 15 minutes seven days a week will theoretically result in only a 0.2-pound weight loss per week, but a 10-pound loss per year will be achieved if the walking is done every day and if food energy intake remains constant.

- A 15-minute brisk walk uses 100 Kcal of energy.
- 100 Kcal × 7 days = 700 Kcal deficit; 3,500 Kcal per pound of fat; 700/3,500 = 0.2 pound loss per week.
- Walking for 15 minutes seven days a week results in a 0.2-pound loss per week.
- Walking for 15 minutes 365 days a year results in a 10.4-pound loss per year.

Even though physical exercise does not contribute greatly to weight loss, it is absolutely necessary for weight maintenance and good health, and moderate exercise is an important factor in preventing regain after weight is lost.

The opportunity costs of being physically active during leisure time include time, effort, and sometimes money. The value of an alternate activity given up to spend time walking in the park has to be balanced with the health benefits. Costs to join a gym or health club or to purchase fitness equipment may be incurred. Health economists Darius Lakdawalla and Tomas Philipson noted that in earlier agricultural and industrial times, energy expenditure was part of one's work, and people were rewarded for their exercise. Today, physical labor is not always built into daily life, and people must spend time and money for exercise (Variyam 2005).

Metabolic and Genetic Contributions

Complex biological mechanisms involving fat cells, hormones, and neurochemical pathways in the brain regulate the balance between energy input and energy expenditure. Fat cells in the body serve two major functions: They store and release fatty acids ingested from food, and they secrete an array of biologically active molecules including the hormone leptin (Bray and Champagne 2005). Leptin, from the Greek word *leptos*, meaning thin, is a hormone produced by fat cells that are also called adipocytes. The hormone was discovered in the 1990s in genetically obese mice that carried the ob, or obese, gene, which rendered them unable to make any leptin. Leptin thus regulates energy expenditure and food intake in rodents. As the amount of fat stored in adipocytes increases, leptin is released into the bloodstream and signals to the brain that the body has had enough to eat. Absolute leptin deficiency in humans, as in mice, causes severe obesity. These genetic defects are extremely rare in humans. Only about 10 children have been identified worldwide who have the disorder.

The discovery of the fat-regulating hormone was met with great hope that injecting obese patients with leptin could produce weight loss. However, clinical trials conducted in 1999 showed that, even with high doses of leptin, only a small amount of weight was lost. The results also demonstrated that most obese people already have high levels of leptin in their bloodstream. It was suggested that people with obesity are leptin resistant, and injecting more of the hormone simply has no effect (Heymsfield et al. 1999).

Information about hunger and satiety also comes from the gastrointestinal tract, where several peptides signal people and animals to stop or start eating. Ghrelin is one peptide that has received recent attention because, in contrast to other gastrointestinal hormones, it stimulates food intake (Cummings and Shannon 2003).

The brain is a major director in regulation of food intake. It receives and transmits information about hunger and satiety. An interesting discovery made in 2004 was that sleep deprivation enhances the release of peptides that produce hunger (Spiegel et al. 2004). In men allowed to sleep only 4 hours per night for two days, leptin decreased and ghrelin increased when compared with the pattern seen in men who slept for 10 hours on each of the two nights. Is it possible that the epidemic of obesity may be a response to lack of sleep?

Can We Blame Obesity on Our Genes?

The role of genetic determinants of obesity such as the ob (obese) gene and the hormone leptin as a modulator of food intake and energy expenditure are intriguing, but they cannot explain the recent epidemic of obesity. Our human genome has not significantly changed in just a few decades. Genes themselves do not make a person obese or thin. They merely determine which individuals are susceptible to weight gain in response to environmental factors. Genetics loads the gun and the environment pulls the trigger.

Ways Genes Contribute to Obesity

Not all people exposed to an abundant food supply are obese. Furthermore, not all obese people exhibit adverse health consequences. This diversity occurs even among groups of the same racial or ethnic background and within families living in the same environment. The variation in how people respond to the same environmental conditions suggests that genes play a role. A common genetic explanation for the rapid rise in obesity is the "thrifty gene" hypothesis: The same genes that made it easier for our ancestors to survive occasional lack of food are now being challenged by environments in which food is always plentiful.

Ways that genes may influence individual propensity for obesity include poor regulation of appetite or the tendency to overeat, inclination to be sedentary or physically inactive, diminished metabolic ability to use dietary fats as fuel, and capacity to preferentially store body fat. The exact pathways by which these genes exert their effects and interact with environmental factors is unknown. Exploration of candidate genes through genomics (the study of genes, their molecular mechanisms, and their associations with health and disease) is an important area for future research regarding overweight and obesity. Use of family history is a straightforward way for clinicians and public health experts to reduce the impact of obesity now. Family history reflects the genetic background and environmental exposures shared by close relatives. Health care practitioners collect family health histories to identify people at high risk of obesity-related disorders such as diabetes, cardiovascular diseases, and some forms of cancer. Weight loss or prevention of excessive weight gain are especially important in this high-risk group. Although all people should follow a healthful diet and incorporate regular physical activity into their daily routine, health promotion programs to reduce disease associated with obesity are more effective if they are directed to the high-risk groups.

Clearly some genetic factors influence excess weight gain. If weight control were simply a matter of willpower, obesity would not be a problem because few people would choose to be fat.

However, genes are not destiny. Obesity can be prevented or managed in most cases with a combination of diet, physical activity, behavior change, medication, or surgery. Finding the most effective combination of treatments for each individual is the challenge we now face.

Consequences of Overweight and Obesity

Although many Americans view overweight as a body image issue, the real concern is the extent to which overweight and obesity contribute directly to morbidity (disease or illness) and mortality (death) (Patel et al. 2006). A declaration from the Office of the Surgeon General of the United States says, "The primary concern of overweight and obesity is one of health and not appearance" (HHS 2007). As Hippocrates noted centuries ago, scientists today find that life expectancy is reduced by obesity. In 2003, before the U.S. House of Representatives, Surgeon General Richard Carmona said, "I welcome this chance to talk with you about a health crisis affecting every State, every city, every community, and every school across our great Nation. The crisis is obesity. It's the fastest growing cause of death in America" (Carmona 2003).

Individuals who are obese (BMI ≥ 30) have a 10 to 50 percent increased risk of death from all causes compared with healthy-weight individuals (BMI 18.5–24.9), and the risk of death rises with increasing weight. Most of the increased deaths are due to cardiovascular causes (NHLBI 1998). Obesity is associated with about 112,000 excess deaths per year in the U.S. population relative to healthy-weight individuals (Flegal et al. 2005).

Overweight and obesity increase risk for developing more than 35 major diseases, including heart disease; hypertension; type 2 diabetes; respiratory problems; osteoarthritis; gallbladder disease; and cancers of the endometrium, breast, prostate, and colon (NHLBI 1998). Obesity also has serious psychological consequences, such as low self-esteem and clinical depression (Kopelman 2000).

According to NHLBI (1998) report:

- The incidence of heart disease (heart attack, congestive heart failure, sudden cardiac death, and angina or chest pain) is increased in persons who have a BMI of 25 or greater.

- High blood pressure is twice as common in adults who are obese than in those who are at a healthy weight, and obesity is associated with elevated triglycerides (blood fat) and decreased HDL cholesterol ("good cholesterol").
- With a weight gain of 11 to 18 pounds, a person's risk of developing type 2 diabetes increases to twice that of individuals who have not gained weight. More than 80 percent of people with diabetes are overweight or obese.
- Sleep apnea (interrupted breathing while sleeping) is more common in obese persons. Obesity is associated with a higher prevalence of asthma.
- For every 2-pound increase in weight, the risk of developing arthritis is increased by 9 to 13 percent. Symptoms of arthritis often improve with weight loss.

Overweight and obesity are associated with an increased risk for some types of cancer, including endometrial (cancer of the lining of the uterus), colon, gallbladder, prostate, kidney, and breast cancer. Women who gain more than 20 pounds after age 18 double their risk of postmenopausal breast cancer, compared with women whose weight remains stable (NHLBI 1998).

Reproductive complications are increased with excess weight. Obesity during pregnancy is linked to increased risk of death in both the baby and the mother. The risk of maternal high blood pressure increases by 10 times for overweight women. Women who are obese during pregnancy are more likely to have gestational diabetes (a form of type 2 diabetes that ceases when the baby is born). Women who are obese during pregnancy are more likely to have high–birth weight infants and may face a higher rate of Cesarean section delivery. Obesity during pregnancy is associated with an increased risk of birth defects, including neural tube defects such as spina bifida.

A wide range of other physical and mental health consequences are related to excess weight. Overweight and obesity are associated with increased risks of gallbladder disease, incontinence, and complications during surgery. Obesity can affect quality of life by limiting mobility and decreasing physical endurance.

As little as 5 to 15 percent of total body weight loss in a person who is overweight or obese reduces the risk factors for some diseases, particularly heart disease and diabetes. Weight reduction is especially beneficial if a person has other risk factors, such as smoking, lack of physical activity, or a family history of heart disease (NHLBI 1998).

Discrimination

Obese individuals endure widespread stigma and discrimination in social, academic, and job situations. Negative perceptions of obese persons exist in the workplace. Research surveys indicated that co-workers and employers viewed obese employees as less competent and lacking in self-discipline. These attitudes can have a negative impact on wages, promotions, and hiring for obese employees. Other studies show that obese applicants are less likely to be hired than thinner applicants, despite having identical job qualifications (Brownell 2005).

Multiple forms of weight stigmatization occur in educational settings. Obese students face numerous obstacles, ranging from harassment to rejection by peers at school. Research shows that stigma toward overweight students begins early. Negative attitudes have been reported among preschool children (ages three to five), who said overweight peers were mean, stupid, ugly, unhappy, and lazy and had few friends (Puhl and Brownell 2001).

Weight stigma also exists in health care settings. Obese patients may be reluctant to seek medical care and are more likely to delay important preventive health care services and cancel medical appointments to avoid experiencing weight bias from health care providers. Negative attitudes about overweight patients have been reported by physicians, nurses, dietitians, psychologists, and medical students. Evidence exists that even health care professionals who specialize in the treatment of obesity hold negative attitudes (Schwartz et al. 2003).

Taken together, the consequences of being denied jobs, rejected by peers, or treated inappropriately by health care professionals because of one's weight can have a serious and negative impact on quality of life. This effect can lead to a number of psychological problems that add to physical difficulties. Obesity-related mental health disorders include depression, anxiety, and despair. Given the pervasive nature of weight stigma in U.S. society, transforming attitudes and enforcing laws that prohibit discrimination based on weight are necessary to decrease the problem of bias against obese individuals.

Economic Consequences

Health problems associated with overweight and obesity have a significant economic impact on the U.S. health care system (HHS 2007). Both direct and indirect health care costs are increased. Direct health care costs refer to preventive, diagnostic, and treatment services such as physician visits, medications, and hospital and nursing home care. Indirect costs occur when people are unable to work because of illness or disability and thus do not receive wages (Colditz 1999).

Studies to determine costs of obesity have shown that health care expenditure among both underweight and overweight individuals increases as BMI varies from the healthy weight range. An analysis of more than 16,000 individuals using data from the 1987 National Medical Expenditure Survey confirmed that BMI, either higher or lower than the healthy weight range normal, was related to increased medical expenditures (Heithoff et al. 1997, Finkelstein et al., 2005).

Further studies indicated that increased health care expenditures were largely related to such costly chronic medical conditions as diabetes and hypertension. Studies from Kaiser Permanente, a large national health maintenance organization, support the BMI and health cost relationship (Thompson, et al. 2001). According to one Kaiser analysis of more than 17,000 patients, total excess costs to the health plan from obese participants amounted to $220 million, or about 6 percent of total expenses for all plan members (Quesenberry, Caan, and Jacobson 1998). Costs were increased among obese members for pharmacy services, outpatient services, and inpatient care.

The significant increase in numbers of extremely obese patients (BMI $\geq$ 40) puts additional strains on the health care system. Lifting injuries among physical therapists, nurses, and other health care workers are on the rise. New hospital expenditures are required for special beds, scales, operating tables, and wheelchairs that will accommodate the weight of very heavy patients.

The costs of obesity treatment must be balanced with predicted outcomes. A weight loss of as little as 5 percent produces health benefits such as lowering blood pressure, blood sugar, and triglycerides (the form in which fat is carried in the blood). Such health improvements could offset the costs of obesity therapy over the long term (NHLBI 1998). However, even after weight loss, formerly obese people need routine follow-up as with control of other chronic conditions such as diabetes. Another factor to be weighed is cost reimbursement. Without adequate reimbursement, physicians are hesitant to take on long-term patient obesity management. Some health insurers cover obesity treatment, but the coverage is not widespread. A key question is: Will a large investment in developing and implementing effective obesity treatment and prevention produce a sufficient increase in good health, happiness, and longevity and a decrease in health care costs?

We Live in an Obesogenic Environment

Although one individual might be born with a stronger tendency to gain weight than another, certain circumstances also must be in place to facilitate weight gain. An environment conducive to weight gain has been termed "obesogenic" (Swinburn, Egger, and Raza 1999). Three primary environmental factors of the obesogenic environment contribute to overweight and obesity:

- Eating more food than the body can use
- Too little exercise or activity
- Lifestyles that interfere with healthy eating and activity (Galvez, Frieden, and Landrigan 2003)

The current situation in the United States encourages energy consumption and discourages energy expenditure to the point that people who could have maintained a healthy weight in past decades find it too difficult to do so today. Americans have easy access to a wide variety of good-tasting, inexpensive, calorie-rich foods that are served and marketed in increasingly large portions. Food is everywhere. It can be found in convenience stores, vending machines, gas stations, museums, and even libraries. The fast-food industry provides a combination of convenience, large portions, and low cost. These factors are attractive to many Americans (Variyam 2005). The food industry spends about $11 billion annually on advertising and $22 billion on consumer promotions. As a result, Americans eat more food than ever before—an average increase of more than 300 calories per day since 1985 (Nestle and Jacobson 2000).

On the energy output side, increasing numbers of Americans lead essentially sedentary lives. Many people sit all day at computers and use cars to get to and from work. Even leisure time is spent in sedentary activities such as watching television and shopping, communicating, or playing games on a computer.

The obesity epidemic is a result of these interacting issues. The solution lies in changing them at individual, community, governmental, and cultural levels. Interventions that have been suggested to help prevent obesity include mass media campaigns, increased availability of exercise opportunities, taxes on high-fat and high-sugar foods, control of food advertising during children's television programming, and restoration of daily physical activity in schools.

Each intervention has positive and negative aspects that may create conflict and controversy. The following chapters will present issues that frame debates about the causes, assessment, treatment, and prevention of obesity. These explanations and findings are based on scientific research that uncovers answers to current concerns about obesity, including the true impact of an obesogenic environment, the merit of various diets, medications or surgeries, and even the stance that obesity may not actually be a public crisis that requires intervention.

References

American College of Sports Medicine (ACSM). *ACSM's Resource Manual for Guidelines for Exercise Testing and Prescription,* 4th ed. Baltimore: Lippincott Williams & Wilkins, 2001.

American Heart Association (AHA). *A Nation at Risk: Obesity in the United States, a Statistical Sourcebook.* Dallas: American Heart Association and the Robert Wood Johnson Foundation, 2005.

Andersen, R. E., C. J. Crespo, S. J. Bartlett, L. J. Cheskin, and M. Pratt. "Relationship of Physical Activity and Television Watching with Body Weight and Level of Fatness among Children: Results from the Third National Health and Nutrition Examination Survey." *Journal of the American Medical Association* 279, no. 12 (1998): 938–942.

Banting, W. *Letter on Corpulence, Addressed to the Public.* London: Harrison, 1864.

Bolanowski, M., and B. E. Nilsson. "Assessment of Human Body Composition Using Dual-Energy X-Ray Absorptiometry and Bioelectrical Impedance Analysis." *Medical Science Monitor* 7, no. 5 (2001): 1029–1033.

Bray, G. A., and C. M. Champagne. "Beyond Energy Balance: There Is More to Obesity Than Kilocalories." *Journal of the American Dietetic Association* 105, no. 5, Suppl. 1 (2005): S17–S23.

Breslow, L. "Public Health Aspects of Weight Control." *American Journal of Public Health and the Nation's Health* 42, no. 9 (1952): 1116–1120.

Brownell, K. D. "The Chronicling of Obesity: Growing Awareness of Its Social, Economic, and Political Contexts." *Journal of Health Politics, Policy and Law* 30, no. 5 (2005): 955–964.

Carmona, R. "The Obesity Crisis in America." In *Testimony before the Subcommittee on Education Reform Committee on Education and the Workforce United States House of Representatives*, edited by Surgeon General, U.S. Public Health Service. Washington, DC: U.S. Department of Health and Human Services, 2003.

Centers for Disease Control and Prevention (CDC). "Portion Size: Then and Now." 2006. [Online information; retrieved 1/5/09.] http://www.cdc.gov/nccdphp/dnpa/nutrition/pdf/portion_size_research.pdf.

Centers for Disease Control and Prevention (CDC). "About BMI for Children and Teens." Atlanta: CDC, 2007a.

Centers for Disease Control and Prevention (CDC). Anthropometric Reference Data, United States, 1988–1994: Centers for Disease Control and Prevention; 1999. [Online information; retrieved 2/5/08.] http://www.cdc.gov/nchs/about/major/nhanes/anthropometric_measures.htm.

Centers for Disease Control and Prevention (CDC). "U.S. Obesity Trends 1985–2006." Atlanta: CDC, 2007b.

Centers for Disease Control and Prevention (CDC). "How Much Physical Activity Do Adults Need?" 2008. [Online information; retrieved 1/29/09.] http://www.cdc.gov/physicalactivity/everyone/guidelines/adults.html.

Colditz, G. A. "Economic Costs of Obesity and Inactivity." *Medicine & Science in Sports & Exercise* 31, no. 11, Suppl. (1999): S663–S667.

Cummings, D. E., and M. H. Shannon. "Roles for Ghrelin in the Regulation of Appetite and Body Weight." *Archives of Surgery* 138, no. 4 (2003): 389–396.

DiMeglio, D. P., and R. D. Mattes. "Liquid versus Solid Carbohydrate: Effects on Food Intake and Body Weight." *International Journal of Obesity and Related Metabolic Disorders* 24, no. 6 (2000): 794–800.

Erselcan, T., F. Candan, S. Saruhan, and T. Ayca. "Comparison of Body Composition Analysis Methods in Clinical Routine." *Annals of Nutrition and Metabolism* 44, no. 5–6 (2000): 243–248.

Finkelstein, E. A., C. J. Ruhm, and K. M. Kosa. "Economic Causes and Consequences of Obesity." *Annual Review of Public Health* 26 (2005): 239–257.

Fisher, J. O., Y. Liu, L. L. Birch, and B. J. Rolls. "Effects of Portion Size and Energy Density on Young Children's Intake at a Meal." *American Journal of Clinical Nutrition* 86, no. 1 (2007): 174–179.

Flegal, K. M., B. I. Graubard, D. F. Williamson, and M. H. Gail. "Excess Deaths Associated with Underweight, Overweight, and Obesity." *Journal of the American Medical Association* 293, no. 15 (2005): 1861–1867.

Ford, E. S., A. H. Mokdad, and W. H. Giles. "Trends in Waist Circumference among U.S. Adults." *Obesity Research* 11, no. 10 (2003): 1223–1231.

Franklin, B. "Poor Richard, an Almanack for 1737." [Online information; retrieved 1/5/09.] http://www.vlib.us/amdocs/index.html.

Gallagher, D. "Overweight and Obesity BMI Cut-offs and Their Relation to Metabolic Disorders in Koreans/Asians." *Obesity Research* 12, no. 3 (2004): 440–441.

Galvez, M. P., T. R. Frieden, and P. J. Landrigan. "Obesity in the 21st Century." *Environmental Health Perspectives* 111, no. 13 (2003): A684–685.

Goran, M. I. "Energy Metabolism and Obesity." *Medical Clinics of North America* 84, no. 2 (2000): 347–362.

Guthrie, J. F., B. H. Lin, and E. Frazao. "Role of Food Prepared Away from Home in the American Diet, 1977–78 versus 1994–96: Changes and Consequences." *Journal of Nutrition Education and Behavior* 34, no. 3 (2002): 140–150.

Guthrie, J. F., and J. F. Morton. "Food Sources of Added Sweeteners in the Diets of Americans." *Journal of the American Dietetic Association* 100, no. 1 (2000): 43–51, quiz 49–50.

Hamwi, G. J. "Therapy: Changing Dietary Concepts." In *Diabetes Mellitus: Diagnosis and Treatment*, edited by T. S. Danowski, 73–78. New York: American Diabetes Association, 1964.

Heithoff, K. A., B. J. Cuffel, S. Kennedy, and J. Peters. "The Association between Body Mass and Health Care Expenditures." *Clinical Therapeutics* 19, no. 4 (1997): 811–820.

Heymsfield, S. B., A. S. Greenberg, K. Fujioka, R. M. Dixon, R. Kushner, T. Hunt, J. A. Lubina, J. Patane, B. Self, P. Hunt, and M. McCamish. "Recombinant Leptin for Weight Loss in Obese and Lean Adults: A Randomized, Controlled, Dose-Escalation Trial." *Journal of the American Medical Association* 282, no. 16 (1999): 1568–1575.

Heymsfield, S. B., Z. Wang, M. Visser, D. Gallagher, and R. N. Pierson, Jr. "Techniques Used in the Measurement of Body Composition: An Overview with Emphasis on Bioelectrical Impedance Analysis." *American Journal of Clinical Nutrition* 64, no. 3, Suppl. (1996): 478S–484S.

Hu, F. B., M. F. Leitzmann, M. J. Stampfer, G. A. Colditz, W. C. Willett, and E. B. Rimm. "Physical Activity and Television Watching in Relation to Risk for Type 2 Diabetes Mellitus in Men." *Archives of Internal Medicine* 161, no. 12 (2001): 1542–1548.

Jakicic, J. M., K. Clark, E. Coleman, J. E. Donnelly, J. Foreyt, E. Melanson, J. Volek, and S. L. Volpe. "American College of Sports Medicine Position Stand. Appropriate Intervention Strategies for Weight Loss and Prevention of Weight Regain for Adults." *Medicine & Science in Sports & Exercise* 33, no. 12 (2001): 2145–2156.

Jakicic, J. M., B. H. Marcus, W. Lang, and C. Janney. "Effect of Exercise on 24-Month Weight Loss Maintenance in Overweight Women." *Archives of Internal Medicine* 168, no. 14 (2008): 1550–1559; discussion 1559–1560.

Johnson, L., A. P. Mander, L. R. Jones, P. M. Emmett, and S. A. Jebb. "Is Sugar-Sweetened Beverage Consumption Associated with Increased Fatness in Children?" *Nutrition* 23, no. 7–8 (2007): 557–563.

Jordan, A. B., J. C. Hersey, J. A. McDivitt, C. D. Heitzler. "Reducing Children's Television-viewing Time: a Qualitative Study of Parents and Their Children." *Pediatrics.* 118, no. 5 (2006): e1303–1310.

Kopelman, P. G. "Obesity as a Medical Problem." *Nature* 404, no. 6778 (2000): 635–643.

Kuczmarski, R. J., and K. M. Flegal. "Criteria for Definition of Overweight in Transition: Background and Recommendations for the United States." *American Journal of Clinical Nutrition* 72, no. 5 (2000): 1074–1081.

Luciano, Lynne. *Looking Good: Male Body Image in Modern America.* New York: Hill and Wang, 2001.

McCrory, M. A., P. J. Fuss, N. P. Hays, A. G. Vinken, A. S. Greenberg, and S. B. Roberts. "Overeating in America: Association between Restaurant Food Consumption and Body Fatness in Healthy Adult Men and Women Ages 19 to 80." *Obesity Research* 7, no. 6 (1999): 564–751.

Metropolitan Life Insurance Company (MLIC). "Metropolitan Life Insurance Company. Ideal Weights for Men 1942." *Statistical Bulletin–Metropolitan Life Insurance Company* 23 (1942): 6–8.

Metropolitan Life Insurance Company (MLIC). "Metropolitan Life Insurance Company. Ideal Weights for Women." *Statistical Bulletin–Metropolitan Life Insurance Company* 24 (1943): 6–8.

Metropolitan Life Insurance Company (MLIC). "New Weight Standards for Men and Women." *Statistical Bulletin–Metropolitan Life Insurance Company* 40 (1959): 1–10.4

Metropolitan Life Insurance Company (MLIC). "1983 Metropolitan Height and Weight Tables: New York." *Statistical Bulletin–Metropolitan Life Insurance Company* 64 (1983): 6–8.

National Center for Health Statistics (NCHS). "Chartbook on Trends in the Health of Americans. Health, United States, 2006." Washington, DC: U.S. Public Health Service, 2006.

Nestle, M., and M. F. Jacobson. "Halting the Obesity Epidemic: A Public Health Policy Approach." *Public Health Reports* 115, no. 1 (2000): 12–24.

National Heart, Lung and Blood Institute (NHLBI). *Clinical Guidelines on the Identification, Evaluation, and Treatment of Overweight and Obesity in Adults: The Evidence Report.* Bethesda, MD: National Heart, Lung and Blood Institute, 1998.

Nielsen, S. J., and B. M. Popkin. "Patterns and Trends in Food Portion Sizes, 1977–1998." *Journal of the American Medical Association* 289, no. 4 (2003): 450–453.

National Institutes of Health (NIH). "Clinical Guidelines on the Identification, Evaluation, and Treatment of Overweight and Obesity in Adults—the Evidence Report. National Institutes of Health." *Obesity Research* 6, Suppl. 2 (1998): 51S–209S.

Olshansky, S. J., D. J. Passaro, R. C. Hershow, J. Layden, B. A. Carnes, J. Brody, L. Hayflick, R. N. Butler, D. B. Allison, and D. S. Ludwig. "A Potential Decline in Life Expectancy in the United States in the 21st Century." *New England Journal of Medicine* 352, no. 11 (2005): 1138–1145.

Patel, M. R., M. Donahue, P. W. Wilson, and R. M. Califf. "Clinical Trial Issues in Weight-Loss Therapy." *American Heart Journal* 151, no. 3 (2006): 633–642.

Powell, L. M., G. Szczypka, F. J. Chaloupka, and C. L. Braunschweig. "Nutritional Content of Television Food Advertisements Seen by Children and Adolescents in the United States." *Pediatrics* 120, no. 3 (2007): 576–583.

Puhl, R., and K. D. Brownell. "Bias, Discrimination, and Obesity." *Obesity Research* 9, no. 12 (2001): 788–805.

Putnam, J., L. S. Kantor, and J. Allshouse. "Per Capita Food Supply Trends: Progress toward Dietary Guidelines " *Food Review* 23 (2000): 2–14.

Quesenberry, C. P., Jr., B. Caan, and A. Jacobson. "Obesity, Health Services Use, and Health Care Costs among Members of a Health Maintenance Organization." *Archives of Internal Medicine* 158, no. 5 (1998): 466–472.

Razak, F., S. S. Anand, H. Shannon, V. Vuksan, B. Davis, R. Jacobs, K. K. Teo, M. McQueen, and S. Yusuf. "Defining Obesity Cut Points in a Multiethnic Population." *Circulation* 115, no. 16 (2007): 2111–2118.

Rolls, B. J., E. L. Morris, and L. S. Roe. "Portion Size of Food Affects Energy Intake in Normal-Weight and Overweight Men and Women." *American Journal of Clinical Nutrition* 76, no. 6 (2002): 1207–1213.

Schwartz, M. B., H. O. Chambliss, K. D. Brownell, S. N. Blair, and C. Billington. "Weight Bias among Health Professionals Specializing in Obesity." *Obesity Research* 11, no. 9 (2003): 1033–1039.

Spiegel, K., E. Tasali, P. Penev, and E. Van Cauter. "Brief Communication: Sleep Curtailment in Healthy Young Men Is Associated with Decreased Leptin Levels, Elevated Ghrelin Levels, and Increased Hunger and Appetite." *Annals of Internal Medicine* 141, no. 11 (2004): 846–850.

Swinburn, B., G. Egger, and F. Raza. "Dissecting Obesogenic Environments: The Development and Application of a Framework for Identifying and Prioritizing Environmental Interventions for Obesity." *Preventive Medicine* 29, no. 6, Pt. 1 (1999): 563–570.

Symonds, Brandreth. "The Influence of Overweight and Underweight on Vitality." *A Weekly Journal of Medicine and Surgery* 74 (1908): 389–393.

Thompson, D., J. B. Brown, G. A. Nichols, P. J. Elmer, and G. Oster. "Body Mass Index and Future Healthcare Costs: a Retrospective Cohort Study." *Obesity Research* 9, no. 3 (2001): 210–218.

U.S. Department of Health and Human Services (HHS). "Overweight and Obesity: Health Consequences." Washington, DC: HHS, 2007.

U.S. Department of Health and Human Services (HHS). "The Surgeon General's Call to Action to Prevent and Decrease Overweight and Obesity."Washington, DC: HHS, 2001.

Variyam, Jayachandran N. "The Price Is Right: Economics and the Rise in Obesity." *Amber Waves* February (2005): 21–27.

Wang, J., J. C. Thornton, S. Kolesnik, and R. N. Pierson, Jr. "Anthropometry in Body Composition. An Overview." *Annals of the New York Academy of Sciences* 904 (2000): 317–326.

Wansink, B., and J. Kim. "Bad Popcorn in Big Buckets: Portion Size Can Influence Intake as Much as Taste." *Journal of Nutrition Education and Behavior* 37, no. 5 (2005): 242–245.

Weight-control Information Network (WIN). "Understanding Adult Obesity." 2006. [Online information; retrieved 1/5/09.] http://win.niddk.nih.gov/publications/understanding.htm.

Wing, R. R. "Physical Activity in the Treatment of the Adulthood Overweight and Obesity: Current Evidence and Research Issues." *Medicine & Science in Sports & Exercise* 31, no. 11, Suppl. (1999): S547–S552.

2

Problems, Controversies, and Solutions

Some of the problems, controversies, and solutions discussed in this chapter have been debated by researchers, health care professionals, and policy makers for many years. Is obesity a disease, or is it a moral failing? Can obesity be called an epidemic? How is obesity treated? The answers to these questions are not simple and have major implications for U.S. society and its health care system.

Is Obesity a Disease?

Advocates of defining obesity as a disease contend that this label will cause the issue to be taken more seriously. Those opposed to calling obesity a disease say it will override personal and societal responsibility. Although not without controversy, increasing scientific evidence and medical consensus support the disease designation. It is generally accepted that a disease must have at least two of the following three features: (1) recognized etiologic agents, (2) identifiable signs and symptoms, and (3) consistent anatomical alterations. Obesity meets all three criteria.

First, the recognized etiologic (causative) agents are a combination of metabolic, physiologic, genetic, social, behavioral, and cultural factors. Second, the identifiable signs and symptoms include an excess accumulation of fat tissue as well as increased risk of breathing problems (sleep apnea), high blood glucose (type 2 diabetes), and abnormal cholesterol level (cardiovascular diseases). Third, the consistent anatomic alteration is a body composition with a high percentage of body fat. Behaviors such as overeating or lack of exercise are not part of the definition of obesity.

Doctors and scientists who say obesity should be labeled as a disease point to its link with increased morbidity and mortality. Physicians who specialize in endocrinology, family practice, and bariatrics accept that obesity is a disease. As a disease, obesity will be the focus of scientists who will have a chance to receive more funding to develop effective interventions. Patients will be able to get the treatment they need, and third-party payers will pay for weight-reduction services. At present, physicians complain that weight management care and counseling services are difficult to code for payment. Without proper coding, they cannot bill for obesity; rather, they have to bill for osteoarthritis, hypertension, diabetes, or other conditions that exist as a side effect of obesity. Most diseases, such as heart disease, cancer, and stroke, are at least partly caused by both lifestyle choices and genetic predisposition. Obesity is the result of a combination of poor lifestyle and genetics in the same way that lung cancer can be the end result of the act of smoking interacting with a genetic predisposition.

Current understanding is that the genetic tendency to obesity is both metabolic and behavioral. Obesity occurs as the result of disturbances in the way energy is stored or expended and of biologically driven abnormalities in appetite, satiation, and satiety. Independent of willpower, a person with one of these disturbances may never be satisfied after eating. Genes, and not personal control, may ultimately determine how much a person eats. Lean individuals may simply be genetically lucky.

Skeptical opponents of calling obesity a disease offer other explanations. They assert that obesity-associated disorders are not necessarily caused by increased body weight. Rather, they propose that a particular disease or treatment for disease may actually promote obesity. These skeptics point to the example of type 2 diabetes, a disorder that currently seems to pose the biggest threat to public health in that some diabetes drugs and strict blood sugar management cause weight gain. Compared with 31 percent prevalence of obesity in the general population, the Centers for Disease Control and Prevention (CDC) reports that 55 percent of adults with diabetes are obese. As obesity has become more prevalent, so has diabetes.

What is the cause, and what is the effect? Does obesity cause diabetes, for example, or does diabetes lead to obesity? Poor health consequences may occur in obese people because they are more likely to belong to an unhealthy group—one that is older or has low socioeconomic status—or to an ethnic minority that has an increased risk for disease in individuals of all weights. Others suggest that it is hazardous weight loss practices and repeated loss and regain of weight that is the major contributor to obesity-related disease (Ernsberger 1989).

Opponents to the disease designation further contend that not all obese people are unhealthy and that calling obesity a medical problem reduces individual responsibility for maintaining a healthy weight. Patients will inevitably have excuses for not taking ownership for their lifestyle habits. Even when people have a genetic tendency to gain weight, overeating and inactivity are the main causes of obesity. The gene pool has not changed, but eating habits have. Some physicians who work with obesity issues also believe obesity is a serious problem, but not a disease in its own right. They say that when obesity is considered a disease it implies that individuals have no control over what is happening to their weight and health. The subject has been a matter of debate for several years among American Medical Association (AMA) members. The AMA continues to recognize obesity as a major public health threat that requires great attention; however, it does not classify obesity as a disease. Among some practitioners there is doubt that applying the label will ensure insurance reimbursement.

Obesity treatment got a boost in 2002 when the Internal Revenue Service recognized obesity as a disease and allowed payments for medically valid obesity treatments to be claimed as a medical tax deduction (IRS 2002). This decision helps to legitimize the possibility of coverage from government and private insurers. Then, in July 2004, U.S. Department of Health and Human Services (HHS) Secretary Tommy Thompson and Medicare administrator Mark McClellan announced that the phrase "Obesity itself cannot be considered an illness" had been removed from regulations that guide payment for medical treatment (HHS 2004). However, the wording change did not authorize any coverage for new treatments. For obesity to be recognized and covered, the provider must first supply scientific evidence that a treatment works to improve Medicare beneficiaries' health outcomes. In other words, practitioners and government and industry partners who believe that obesity is an actual disease are responsible for collecting data from clinical trials on the effectiveness of proposed treatments. The results will be ready to present when the agency is prepared to review them. As with the public health response to smoking, government regulation and changes in behavior, both voluntary and mandated (such as the restriction on smoking in public places) will be extensively debated before any policy is formulated. Of course, the two health issues differ greatly in that individuals do not have to smoke to live but must eat to survive.

Considerable debate also surrounds how the disease label will affect individual patients with regard to stigma. Proponents maintain that diagnosing obesity as a serious disease removes the stigma associated with extra body fat. Those opposed argue that the disease designation actually further stigmatizes people who do not feel sick and do not notice any ill effects from extra weight. This line of thinking underscores one of the problems surrounding efforts to address obesity: An unhealthy diet and a sedentary lifestyle are health risks for anyone—fat or lean. Thus, those opposed to the disease label are concerned that reclassifying obesity as a disease places too much emphasis on the number on the scale and neglects the importance of a healthful lifestyle. As even the best weight loss interventions have limited efficacy, telling a patient to lose weight generally results in frustration and guilt. Many clinicians propose alternative strategies such as encouraging the individual to eat more fruits and vegetables, to get adequate sleep, and to enjoyable physical activity. These changes might actually prolong and improve life for all sizes.

Defining obesity as a disease may put too much emphasis on the medical aspect when every institution and individual involved should accept some responsibility. A number of businesses are taking on that responsibility. Food companies are pledging to make healthier snacks. Fast-food chains promise new low-fat choices. Employers are integrating health management options such as gyms, diet groups, cafeterias with healthful foods, and health screening right at the work site. Health plans and doctors are initiating new prevention, treatment, and weight-management programs. Local communities are constructing more walking and bike trails and after-school-activity programs for children.

In summing up the pros and cons of whether obesity is a disease, those who agree say:

- Obesity is linked to increased morbidity and mortality.
- Everyone would take the condition more seriously.
- There would be better reimbursement for medical treatment.
- Obese people would not be stigmatized as lacking willpower.

Those who disagree say:

- It would reduce the importance of individual responsibility.
- It would place too much emphasis on medical interventions.
- It would put undue social pressure and stigma on obese people who are healthy.
- The evidence is not sufficient to implicate obesity as a risk factor in its own right. (Stagg-Elliott 2006)

Is Obesity an Epidemic?

A public opinion survey found that 85 percent of Americans believe that obesity is an epidemic and that the government should have a role in tackling the obesity crisis (Levi, Segal, and Gadola 2007). In 2001, U.S. Surgeon General David Satcher declared that obesity was reaching epidemic proportions and could soon be the cause of as much preventable disease and death as cigarette smoking. He released a call to action to promote the recognition of obesity as a health problem and to develop programs to treat obesity and encourage people to change their eating and exercise habits. But even with the urging of America's top physician, obesity statistics did not improve and the rate of overweight and obesity kept growing. As quoted in Chapter 1, at a congressional briefing in 2003, Surgeon General Richard H. Carmona spoke about the obesity crisis in the United States—it bears repeating here: "As Surgeon General, I welcome this chance to talk with you about a health crisis affecting every State, every city, every community, and every school across our great nation. The crisis is obesity. It is the fastest-growing cause of disease and death in America."

He goes on to say, "And it is completely preventable. Nearly two out of every three Americans are overweight or obese. One out of every eight deaths in America is caused by an illness directly related to overweight and obesity" (Carmona 2003).

"Epidemic" is an emotionally charged term. It has different meanings for different people. For the general public, it is associated with a rapidly spreading and uncontrolled disease. Professional health researchers may use the term quite differently. Epidemiologists define an epidemic as the occurrence in a specified area of an illness or other health-related events in excess of what would normally be expected. Disease and epidemics occur as a result of the interaction of three factors: agent, host, and environment. Agents (too much food) cause the disease (extra body fat), hosts are genetically susceptible, and environmental conditions (easy access to high-calorie foods and reduced need to be active) permit host exposure to the agent. Understanding interactions between agent, host, and environment is crucial for discovering the best ways to prevent or control the spread of obesity.

Obesity has been called an epidemic in the United States because one-third of Americans are obese and two-thirds are overweight or obese. Looking at state-by-state statistics, one can see how the prevalence of obesity seems to spread and grow each year. (See Figure 6.1 in Chapter 6, showing obesity trends, epidemiologic data, and data that show increasing percentage of obesity by state.) Adult obesity rates increased in 31 states in 2007. Mississippi led the list with the highest rate of adult obesity in the United States. It was the first state to reach an obesity rate of more than 30 percent of the state population. Colorado was the leanest state; however, its adult obesity rate has also slowly and steadily increased over the years. Ten of the states with the highest rates of adult obesity were located in the South (CDC 2007).

The Center for Consumer Freedom (CFF) is a nonprofit organization of restaurants, food companies, and consumers. Its stated goal is to promote personal responsibility and protect consumer choice. The group has published a response to the description of obesity as an epidemic entitled "An Epidemic of Obesity Myths" (CFF 2004). It says the epidemic is a myth because, while more people are heavier than ever, the figures used to calculate the number of deaths attributed to obesity are flawed and the health risks of moderate obesity have been greatly overstated. The Center also contends that better diagnosis and treatment of high cholesterol and blood pressure have more than compensated for any increases in mortality from rising obesity.

CCF may not have been too far off the mark when it pointed out problems with past statistical estimations of obesity-increased risk of death. In 2005, Dr. Katherine Flegal, a researcher at the CDC, revised estimates of the deaths due to obesity after it became clear that previous measurement methods were out-of-date. The new estimate, published in the *Journal of the American Medical Association*, showed that people in the overweight category, with a body mass index (BMI) of 25 to 29.9, typically live longer than normal-weight people, who have a BMI of 18 to 24.9 (Flegal et al. 2005). Flegal and her colleagues reported that the number of obesity-related deaths is significantly lower than previously believed. When National Health and Nutrition Examination Surveys (NHANES) data, which measured weights, heights, and death from 1988 to 2000, were analyzed, even severe obesity failed to appear as a statistically significant mortality risk.

More than a dozen other studies have come to the same conclusion. Epidemiological studies reveal that, aside from the extremes, BMI is not a strong predictor of death rates. The minimum risk for mortality seems to be associated with a BMI of approximately 25. The risk of death increases or decreases on upper or lower side of 25, respectively. Flegal's group speculates that in recent decades, improvements in medical care have reduced the mortality level associated with obesity (Flegal et al. 2005). This speculation is supported by research (also based on NHANES data) showing, in spite of increases in overweight and obesity, significant declines in high blood pressure, high cholesterol, and smoking. These are all risk factors for cardiovascular disease. Importantly, the greatest improvements occurred in the heaviest people (Gregg et al. 2005). Although Americans are heavier than ever, they are also healthier than they were in the 1960s and 1970s. The average BMI was lower in those days, but the rate of deaths from cancer and heart disease was higher. In short, people live longer now (NCHS 2007).

Even though the CDC findings, reported widely in the media, caused confusion and questions about whether obesity really was a problem, some facts about obesity are not disputed. The proportion of the population that is overweight or obese continues to rise rapidly. Despite debates about obesity as a cause of death, there is little argument about the significant impact it has as a cause of disease. Excess weight is known to be a major contributor to diabetes, cardiovascular diseases, arthritis, and some forms of cancer. Even if obesity does cause fewer deaths than have previously been reported, it continues to be a serious public health problem.

An interesting addition to the discussion about whether obesity is an epidemic was published in the *New England Journal of Medicine*. The researchers suggested that obesity is influenced by one's social network and that it is "socially contagious." To see if obesity really did behave like an epidemic, they studied the effects of these groups on obesity. They examined data from the Framingham Heart Study—a very large social network that involves 12,000 people, including family, friends, and neighbors who have been studied and followed for more than 30 years. The results showed that a person's chances of becoming obese increased by 57 percent if she or he had a friend who became obese, by 40 percent if she or he had a sibling who became obese, and by 37 percent if her or his spouse became obese. The infectious effect was greater among friends of the same sex. A 71 percent increased risk of obesity was seen if a same-sex friend became obese (Christakis and Fowler 2007).

Further, a person's chances of becoming obese were influenced by his or her family and friends, even if they were hundreds of miles away. How could this possibly occur? The dramatic effect of distant friends on the odds of increased obesity rules out exposure to the same environment as a cause. The Christakis study analyses revealed that similar weights were not due to any tendency for people to interact with others like them, eating the same foods as their friends did, or participating in the same physical activities as their friends did. It may be that esteem for friends influences a person's conception of a normal, healthy, and attractive body size. The investigators found that thinness also appeared to be socially contagious. When a person lost weight and was no longer obese, her or his friends and family tended to lose weight, too. The scientists proposed that this contagious social influence should be exploited to spread positive health behaviors from one person to the entire social network.

Another remarkable theory about how obesity may occur has been put forth by a group of researchers who have implicated a virus in the development of obesity in animals and possibly in humans. In 1992, Nikhil Dhurandhar, at the University of Bombay, reported that an avian adenovirus—Ad36—caused excessive fat in chickens (Dhurandhar et al. 2000). Researchers began to look for antibodies against this type of virus in obese humans. The presence of antibodies against the virus means that the person had been exposed to the virus at some time. When Richard Atkinson, professor of medicine and nutrition at the University of Wisconsin, Madison, and Dhurandhar screened humans in India and the United States for Ad36 antibodies, they found that approximately 30 percent of the people with obesity had the antibodies, compared with only 10 percent of the normal-weight people (Atkinson et al. 2005). The researchers theorize that the virus somehow affects the brain centers that control appetite. Quoted in *DOC News*, Atkinson said, "We can't say that the virus caused obesity in all those people. It's still speculation, some say a gross speculation (Kolakowski 2005).

Treatment of Obesity: Fighting the Battle of the Bulge

There are no simple solutions to the obesity problem. Obesity is a complex disease that requires complex solutions. Successful treatment of obesity and overweight requires lifelong behavioral changes rather than short-term weight loss or quick fixes. Programs that emphasize realistic goals, gradual progress, sensible eating, and exercise are recommended by weight-loss experts. Those that promise instant weight loss or feature severely restricted diets are not effective in the long run. Unfortunately, the success rate for even sensible diets is approximately 3 to 5 percent. Studies show that most people regain a considerable amount of weight by one year and nearly everyone returns to her or his pre-diet weight after five years (Wadden et al. 1989).

Long-term management of obesity is the most challenging aspect of weight control for many individuals. Whatever method of weight loss is used, the preferred goals of treatment are similar. In the past, physicians and other experts who designed treatment programs encouraged people to achieve their ideal weight based on height-weight charts or recommended BMI. Given the lack of success in preventing weight regain, most programs now aim for the "10 percent solution"—to lose about 10 percent of body weight. The focus is on improving overall health rather than attaining a certain weight.

Attempting to lose weight is a common pursuit for many Americans. A study published in 2005 reported that 46 percent of U.S. women and 33 percent of U.S. men said they were trying to lose weight (Bish et al. 2005). The approaches that most people use typically include a combination of dieting, increasing physical activity, lifestyle modification and behavioral changes. Some dieters try dietary supplements or medications that theoretically could increase or speed up weight loss. For individuals who haven't had success with diet, lifestyle, and medication, various types of surgery may be an option.

For those who enjoy a structure of companionship and support while trying to manage weight, a wide variety of weight-loss groups are available. Do-it-yourself programs include groups like Overeaters Anonymous (OA) and TOPS (Take Off Pounds Sensibly). These self-help groups are free of charge and are led by group members. TOPS advises a low-calorie, low-fat meal plan, while OA encourages members to abstain from refined foods that might act as triggers to overeat. The OA philosophy helps to guide participants to physical, emotional, and spiritual recovery. Minimal scientific evidence is available to examine success rates from these two groups.

Commercial franchises like Weight Watchers, Jenny Craig, and Nutrisystem offer meetings, materials, and even meals. These groups rely on counselors to provide services to clients. In an evaluation of the success of the best-known commercial programs, people who followed the Weight Watchers plan maintained a greater than 5 percent weight loss over 12 months. Participants attending the most group sessions kept off the most weight, clearly showing the importance of staying with the program (Tsai and Wadden 2005).

Clinical programs provided by medical professionals who may have specialized training to treat obese patients focus on medical nutrition therapy, exercise, and psychological counseling. They can feature very-low-calorie diets (VLCDs) and liquid diets, medications, and surgery. Medically supervised proprietary programs, such as Optifast, Health Maintenance Resources, and Medifast, place patients on very-low-calorie, high-protein plans (usually about 800 calories per day). These programs customarily use liquid diets in place of solid food, and participants are closely monitored by a physician. The theory is that a VLCD could be effective for obese individuals to start their weight loss if they have the medical supervision critical for following it safely. Afterward, a transitional period with measured meal replacements, slow reintroduction to foods, and education about new ways of healthy eating should help ensure long-term success. Studies show patients completing these programs can lose approximately 15 to 25 percent of their initial weight during three to six months of treatment and maintain a loss of 8 to 9 percent at one year (Tsai and Wadden 2005). The success rate might be overestimated, as the results did not include those who dropped out of programs. A task force from the National Heart, Lung and Blood Institute (NHLBI) has indicated that one year after the diet is completed, VLCDs do not result in any greater weight reduction when compared with other, less stringent diets providing 1,200 to 1,500 calories (NHLBI 1998).

Several commercial Internet-based programs offer meal plans, recipes, online chats with other dieters, and e-mail advice from experts such as dietitians and psychologists. Published evidence of outcomes from eDiets showed participants losing 1.1 percent of their initial weight after one year. This type of information and support could be used on its own or could supplement other programs. The convenience of online record keeping of daily intake and activity could possibly increase weight maintenance.

The struggle to lose unwanted pounds requires choosing between responsible products and programs that offer methods for achieving moderate weight loss over time and "miracle" products or services that promise fast and easy weight loss without sacrifice. Advertisements for weight-loss products and services flood the marketplace with promises of instant success without the need to give up favorite foods or increase physical activity. An example of such an eye-grabbing ad reads, "Amazing New Discovery, Guarantees Weight-Loss, Eliminates Dieting ... And Can Slash Up To 29 Pounds Of Embarrassing Fat From Your Body Almost Overnight—Without Wasting 1 Minute Of your Day!" as seen on the Internet at get-slim-while-you-sleep. com. Almost all weight-loss experts agree that the key to long-term weight management requires permanent lifestyle changes that include a healthful diet at a moderate calorie level and regular physical exercise. Nevertheless, only about one in three people reported trying to lose weight by eating less and engaging in the minimum recommended amount of physical activity (30 minutes on most, preferably all, days of the week). Even fewer —about one in four people—followed the approach recommended in the *Dietary Guidelines for Americans 2005* of eating less and engaging in approximately 60 minutes of moderate- to vigorous-intensity activity on most days of the week (about 300 or more minutes per week).

A large gap remains between recommended dietary patterns and what Americans actually eat. Only 3 percent of all individuals in the United States meet the dietary goal for daily intake of whole grains, fruits, and vegetables.

With dozens of new diets and miraculous foods being advertised, people find it hard to know what to eat, what to avoid, and whom to believe. For a healthy diet beneficial both for weight loss and for improving long-term health, the U.S. Department of Agriculture's (USDA) *Dietary Guidelines for Americans* provides practical examples of healthful diet choices for everyone. Every five years, HHS and USDA jointly publish the *Dietary Guidelines for Americans,* based on the latest scientific evidence. The latest version was released in January 2005. The guidelines exist to provide people with authoritative advice about the most healthful dietary habits. The guidelines also are the basis for federal food and nutrition education programs and are depicted graphically as the Food Guide Pyramid (FGP), which recommends types and amounts of foods from seven food groups—grains, vegetables, fruits, milk, meat and beans, oils, and discretionary calories—as well as physical activity.

The guidelines are not specifically weight loss diets. They are presented across a range of calorie levels for people over two years of age with recommended calorie intake and food patterns for individuals based on age, gender, and activity level. "MyPyramid Calorie Levels" is a chart that shows the appropriate calories needed for males and females by age and activity level. "MyPyramid Food Intake Patterns" identifies suggested amounts of food to consume from the various food groups at 12 different calorie levels. (See Table 6.4 and Table 6.5 in Chapter 6.) The entire set of recommendations is intended to be used in the context of planning an overall healthful diet. However, following *any* of the recommendations can have health benefits.

The FGP has been received with some criticism. Public health advocates, nutritionists, and health care providers indicate that it is not clear or easy to understand. To follow personalized recommendations, the public has to use the pyramid Web site. Information is lacking about what foods may be considered unhealthy, and the guidelines did not receive adequate funding from the federal government to fully promote them.

In spite of these drawbacks, the advice contained in these guidelines related to choosing a variety of healthy foods in correct portions is a good way to maintain a healthy weight. Professional weight-management experts generally use the USDA guidelines in combination with other general strategies to reduce calorie intake. Suggestions for personal weight management often include the following advice:

1. **Make an individualized plan and assessment**. Begin with an evaluation of what you are eating. This is called a current diet assessment. The word "diet" brings to mind meals of tuna and carrot sticks or dry toast. A diet is actually all the food and beverages that a person takes in during the course of a day. People generally underestimate how much they eat and often do not remember what they ate from one day to the next, so keeping a journal that lists actual amounts of all food and beverages consumed can be an effective tool to identify foods that contribute to weight gain. Table 6.6 in Chapter 6 is an example of a form for keeping a record of when one eats, what, and how much one is eating, and the hunger level experienced. Using the program entails matching the foods on the form with daily goals in "MyPyramid Calorie Levels" and "MyPyramid Food Intake Patterns" or using MyPyramid Tracker to assess the quality of one's diet. MyPyramid Tracker is an online, interactive dietary and physical activity assessment tool that translates the principles of the 2005 *Dietary Guidelines for Americans* into individualized healthful choices. Personalized recommendations are made for food and activity depending on one's age, sex, and weight. The Food Calories/Energy Balance feature automatically calculates energy balance by subtracting the energy expended from physical activity from food energy intake. Using this tool helps to point out links between good nutrition and regular physical activity and assists in keeping track of the food and exercise history for up to one year (CNPP 2008).

2. **Reduce energy intake**. A 500- to 1,000-calorie-per-day deficit can result in a weight loss of 1 to 2 pounds of fat

per week. This type of energy reduction is designed to achieve slow, progressive weight loss, and for most people this means that the reduced energy plan will total about 1,000 to 1,200 calories for women and 1,200 to 1,600 calories for men. The MyPyramid online tools provide a good guide to meal plans for these calorie levels. Even with some guidelines, evaluating calorie content of foods takes practice because energy content is not always obvious. For a woman with a goal of 1,200 calories per day, just six chocolate sandwich cookies provide more than one-quarter of those calories. Calorie content of foods can be estimated using online databases, food labels, restaurant nutrition information sheets, and handbooks of nutrient information.

3. **Recognize fat as a concentrated source of energy.** Fat is a concentrated source of calories. It has 9 calories per gram, whereas protein and carbohydrate have only 4 calories per gram. Thus, fat can supply more than twice as many calories in each bite as a bite of carbohydrate or protein. In a given weight of food, the most efficient way to reduce calories is to cut back on the fat. In the campaign to prevent obesity, the NHLBI suggests limiting total fat to 30 percent or less of total calories. For example, in a 2,000-calorie diet, about 660 calories—or about 75 grams of fat—could come from fat in meals each day. Studies show that people consume more total energy with high-fat diets compared with low fat diets (NHLBI 1998).

4. **Eat less fat and sugar and more fruits and vegetables.** Calorie density of menu items can be diluted by the addition of fruits, vegetables, whole grains, and water. For example, extra vegetables and whole grain bread can reduce the calorie density of a meat sandwich. Plant fiber adds volume and provides a feeling of fullness, so fewer overall calories may be consumed.

5. **Limit food quantity at home and when eating out.** By recalibrating portion sizes to fit individual health goals, it is possible to eat all types of foods in moderation at home or when eating out. Even without measuring spoons or cups, the amount of a standard food portion may be visualized by comparison to objects of similar size. For example, three ounces of meat or poultry is about the size of a deck of cards or the palm of one's

hand. One-half cup of cooked rice, pasta, or potato is similar in size to half of a baseball or the amount that can fit in a cupped hand. A serving size card with more examples of what one serving looks like can be downloaded at http://hp2010.nhlbihin.net/portion/keep.htm.

Dozens of complex diets have been promoted for weight loss, but there is no scientific evidence to show that any one diet is more effective than another. Table 6.7 in Chapter 6 helps sort through the various types of diets that exist today. It lists some of the most common diet plans, examines their advantages and disadvantages, and provides the dietary basis behind their potential benefits.

Currently, there is considerable interest in the effects of individual macronutrients—fat, protein, and carbohydrate—to make weight management easier or more effective. High-carbohydrate, high-fiber, low-fat diets like those proposed by Dean Ornish and Nathan Pritikin include whole grains, fruits, and vegetables. These diets limit all types of dietary fat. Fat is not intrinsically bad, but because fat contains twice the calories of protein or carbohydrate, reduced-fat meals provide more food volume for fewer calories.

High-fat, high-protein, low-carbohydrate food plans, such as the Atkins diet, may be more satisfying than low-fat diets. With this approach, less food could be eaten, but weight loss does not occur unless fewer calories are consumed overall. A review of nearly 100 studies of low-carbohydrate weight loss diets did not find enough evidence to recommend for or against the use of such diets. Weight loss was related to eating fewer calories and staying on the diet for a longer period of time, but not with the carbohydrate content of food (Bravata et al. 2003). At this time, no reliable data are available to show that any combination or avoidance of foods will work better than the others over the long term. The closer a person follows any calorie-reduced diet, the greater the weight loss. It is the adherence to a diet, not the diet itself, that makes the difference (Bray and Champagne 2005). No one intervention works equally for everyone. Not everybody loses weight. Of those who do so, the majority are unable to keep it off. Before experts are able to predict that diet plans will actually cause weight loss for longer than six months, they need more data about matching the diet intervention to individual metabolic and social needs.

Diet Foods

The U.S. food and beverage industries have launched massive campaigns to develop and promote reduced-calorie foods using products such as artificial sweeteners and fat replacers. It is not certain how these foods contribute to weight management for most Americans. Do people actually lose weight by snacking on fat-free chips and sugar-free pudding? Perhaps they just feel free to eat more of everything. Although it seems to make sense that exchanging high-calorie sweeteners with sugar-free substitutes could help control weight, no scientific consensus has been reached regarding their value. In a review of laboratory, clinical, and epidemiological studies, artificial sweeteners were associated with only modest weight loss (Bellisle and Drewnowski 2007). The sweeteners did not suppress appetite or further consumption of food. It was suggested that they could only be a benefit if they were integrated into a reduced-calorie diet. Although some investigators have concluded that artificial sweeteners enhance weight loss, others have suggested that they actually increase body weight. This idea is based on studies such as one in France that showed that people who regularly consume artificial sweeteners have a higher BMI (West and de Looy 2001). Instead of suggesting a causal relationship between artificial sweeteners and increased body weight, these data may reflect practices in which individuals were using artificial sweeteners to reduce calories because they were already overweight. Little is known about the long-term impact of sweetener replacements on energy intake and body weight.

The American Heart Association and the American Dietetic Association report that fat substitutes can have a substantial impact on weight reduction as long as they lower total calorie intake (Wylie-Rosett 2002). Olestra (which goes by the brand name Olean) is a synthetic mixture of sugar and vegetable oil that passes through the body undigested. Olestra-based foods have the sensory qualities of real fat; however, concern has been expressed about its safety based on reports from individuals who experienced gastrointestinal problems, such as cramps and loose stools, after consuming large amounts of olestra. Olestra has been studied more than many other fat substitutes, and a review of more than 100 studies has shown that consumption of olestra-containing food does not affect gastric emptying or bowel transit times. Occurrence of gastrointestinal symptoms under ordinary snacking conditions with olestra is similar to those that occur following consumption of snacks fried in regular fats. Olestra does cause a decrease in the availability of fat-soluble vitamins A, D, E, and K, but this deficit is offset by the U.S. Food and Drug Administration (FDA)–mandated addition of these vitamins to olestra-containing foods (Hunt, Zorich, and Thomson 1998; Thomson, Hunt, and Zorich 1998).

Several studies on the effects of olestra on appetite and energy intake showed that replacement of dietary fat with olestra resulted in weight loss that was significantly greater than a control diet. In these studies, weight loss occurred because total energy intake was reduced. The overall results from studies of sugar and fat replacers and increased dietary fiber indicate that some products used to reduce energy density are helpful in obesity management, while others do not make a significant contribution. The essential factor that determines effectiveness of modified food products is that total energy in a person's meals and snacks must be decreased, or the benefit of energy-reduced foods for weight management is limited (Bray et al. 2004).

Nutritionists caution the public to be aware of the realities of the weight-reduction potential of reduced-calorie foods and not buy completely into the promises (Kazaks and Stern 2008). The realities are that calories do count. Calories consumed must equal calories expended even with low-energy-density foods. A reduced-calorie food label is not a license to eat unlimited amounts guilt free. Low-calorie products should be used as substitutes for higher-calorie foods, not in addition to a regular diet. Furthermore, lower-calorie foods should taste good. Not all products provide desirable flavors, aromas, and textures. The promises of successful weight management by reduced-calorie food consumption is based on the theory that following a reduced-calorie diet is easier when the taste and qualities of sugars and fats are provided in reduced-calorie versions of foods. It is anticipated that the volume of food in low-calorie, high-fiber products may help consumers be satisfied with smaller portions at each meal and, consequently, fewer calories overall.

Adequate Nutrition Labeling

Nutrition labels can help consumers make the informed food choices that contribute to a healthy diet. In 1990, the Nutrition Labeling and Education Act (NLEA) was signed into law. This act was a new mandate for food manufacturers to disclose the fat (saturated and unsaturated), cholesterol, sodium, sugar, fiber, protein, and carbohydrate content in their products. It required retailers to provide labels for their store's 20 top-selling fruits, vegetables, fish, and shellfish, although meat, poultry and egg products, infant formula, foods sold in bulk, foods with insignificant amounts of nutrients, and foods sold by retailers with total sales of less than $500,000 were exempt from the requirement. Retailers did not have to label each item, but if they chose not to, they were required to provide this information in a single location in the store.

In 1993, the FDA and the USDA issued regulations that specified the table format and content of nutrition labels on most foods, including processed meat and poultry products. The nutrition facts table is intended to contain easy-to-read and easy-to-use information that allows purchasers to understand the nutritional value of a food, compare products, and increase or decrease consumption of nutrients or calories. More resources related to the nutrition facts label may be found in Chapter 7; see also "How to Understand and Use the Nutrition Facts Label" at http://www.cfsan.fda.gov/~dms/foodlab.html.

Although consumers have the right to nutrition information about food products, NLEA did not cover foods purchased in restaurants and at prepared food counters in grocery stores. Despite the fact that people are eating more food away from home, usually they can only guess at the calorie content of the items they order. Most restaurants have no trouble listing the price of menu items, but only about a third provide nutrition information on the menus. Without having the information right where the food purchasing decision is made, most people have difficulty comparing options and making the most healthful choice. A study conducted in 2006 with more than 5,000 Americans who answered questionnaires about their food purchases revealed that, on average, they ate away from home about six times per week. In that study consumers agreed that they were ultimately responsible for making sensible food choices; however, 41 percent wanted to see more nutrition information printed on menus so they could choose well (Malone and Bland-Campbell 2005). The Institute of Medicine, FDA, Office of the Surgeon General, and AMA all called for prominently visible displays of calories and other nutrition information at the point of choice in restaurant chains. The Center for Science in the Public Interest, a consumer advocate group whose goals are to counter the food industry's influence on public opinion and public policies and to lobby for government policies, was at the forefront of efforts to make calorie content of purchased food readily available.

In 2006, the New York City Department of Health and Mental Hygiene became the first agency to require most restaurants to show calorie information on menus and menu boards. In 2007, the New York State Restaurant Association (NYSRA) challenged the regulation and it was subsequently blocked. The Department of Health loosened some of the rules that the NYSRA had objected to and reinstated the menu-labeling regulation. A subsequent motion filed by chain restaurant lobbyists to again block the requirement that the calorie value of dishes must be displayed alongside prices was rejected by a U.S. District Court judge. The judge agreed with the argument that showing calorie values alongside prices will help consumers make choices that will lead to a lower incidence of obesity, and the regulation went into effect in 2008. The judge's ruling meant that any restaurant chain with 15 or more nationwide outlets, or about 10 percent of the restaurants in the boroughs of New York City —Manhattan, Brooklyn, Queens, the Bronx, and Staten Island— are required to display calorie counts on menus, menu display boards, and food tags. Advocates of menu labeling say this landmark decision paves the way for other local and state governments to pass similar measures.

Physical Activity

As discussed previously, moderate exercise does not greatly contribute to weight reduction. Exercise does use up calories, and the cumulative effects of regular exercise over long periods of time can be beneficial in preventing weight gain. However, calorie expenditure from low-level activity is not adequate to permit increased food intake. When individuals have unrealistic expectations that exercise can increase weight loss, they may become disappointed at the lack of results. The true benefits of exercise are preventing weight gain, decreasing body fat, maintaining weight loss, and improving general health at any weight. For long-term good health, an important goal is to establish a regular, sustained pattern of physical activity (Wadden and Foster 2000).

Behavioral Strategies for Responding to an Obesogenic Environment

Living in an obesogenic environment—one that encourages sedentary living and aggressively promotes consumption of high-energy-density foods—requires increasing effort to overcome this barrier to good health. Behavioral treatment of overweight and obesity trains individuals to gain control over unhealthful external conditions as they identify and modify personal dietary and physical activity responses that lead to overweight.

Four behavioral strategies commonly applied to weight loss and maintenance programs are (1) self-monitoring, (2) stimulus control, (3) cognitive restructuring, and (4) social support (Fujioka 2002).

1. **Self-monitoring diet and exercise patterns**: To change behaviors, it helps people to become aware of their actions such as overeating or being sedentary. Keeping a journal listing all food and beverages consumed and the duration and frequency of physical activity can be an effective learning tool because it pinpoints the amounts and types of food eaten and exercise performed each day. Daily food and activity records provide immediate feedback, so a problem pattern becomes obvious and possible solutions can be tried right away. Self-monitoring data can be recorded in a diary or notebook, as entries into a handheld computer, or with the use of a computerized diet and exercise analysis program. Exercise can be monitored in time or distance, as with the use of a pedometer. People generally underestimate how much they eat and overreport exercise. Record keeping decreases the tendency of both lean and obese people to underestimate their food intake (Kretsch, Fong, and Green 1999). Reducing energy intake is the key to weight reduction, and accurate assessment of food intake by keeping food records is consistently related to weight loss (NHLBI 1998).

2. **Stimulus control**: Personal diet and activity records can identify the "triggers," or environmental cues associated

with incidental eating, overeating, and inactivity. Generally, weight-management guides, diet books, and Web sites provide a wide variety of tips or ideas for managing cues.

3. **Cognitive restructuring—defining weight loss success**: If dieters are to develop reasonable weight-loss goals, they must correct false beliefs and expectations. Most dieters have unrealistic ideas about the amount of weight they want to lose and the extent of weight loss that is possible with even the best treatment. Instead of aiming for ideal weight based on the Metropolitan Life Insurance Company's height-weight charts, people should target a 10 percent reduction in body weight, as suggested above, for a successful outcome. Losing as little as 5–10 percent of initial weight has been shown to improve hypertension, type 2 diabetes, and abnormal cholesterol levels, even if the person is not at ideal body weight (NHLBI 1998). Most individuals expect that dieting will result in much more weight lost than these modest goals. A study published in 2000 reported that participants who lost 10 percent of their body weight during a four-month treatment were disappointed and felt that they had failed because their weight loss was not, to them, sufficient (Foster et al. 2001). In this study, nearly 400 women beginning a weight-loss program were asked to describe their goal weight loss in terms of what they wished to achieve, what they would be happy with, and weight loss they would view as unsuccessful. The women said they aimed for about a 38 percent reduction in body weight—more than three times the recommended goal. A 25 percent reduction was described as just "acceptable," but not one they would be happy with. A 16 percent loss was considered "disappointing." These responses suggest that many dieters have unrealistic goals and, even after a medically significant weight loss, they may feel unsuccessful (Foster et al. 2001). Cognitive restructuring is also useful in dealing with lapses or weight regain. Individuals are encouraged to see the setback for what it is—a temporary lapse from which it is possible to recover, instead of total failure. The setback is assessed to determine why the lapse occurred and how a similar situation could be prevented in the future. Other

techniques include rehearsing ways to cope with relapse before it occurs. Each time a challenge is successfully managed—even an imaginary one—the chances of relapse are reduced (Wadden and Foster 2000).

4. **Social support network**: People with a social support network are more successful at weight loss and maintenance than those without strong support systems. Sixty-six percent of women who participated in behavior modification groups along with friends were able to maintain total weight loss 10 months after treatment compared with only 24 percent of those in the group of people who were recruited alone (Wing 1999). Scientific literature on weight maintenance of greater than three years shows that diet combined with group therapy and social support have the best chance of long-term success (Ayyad and Andersen 2000). Most weight is lost during the first six months of treatment (Wadden and Foster 2000). Numerous studies show that weight loss is enhanced by long-term behavioral treatment, but attendance at sessions generally declines over time, and without support and encouragement and having to be accountable for healthful lifestyle choices, people regain weight. For most dieters, about a third of the initial weight loss is regained in the year after treatment. Three to five years later, at least 50 percent of participants have returned to their initial weight or gained more. Behavioral maintenance therapy can delay weight regain, but data are insufficient to prove that it is effective over the long term (Kramer et al. 1989).

Long-term Success

The National Weight Control Registry (NWCR) shows that some people are successful at long-term weight management on their own. The NWCR was a project developed in 1994 by Dr. Rena Wing and Dr. James Hill to help identify those individuals who have succeeded at long-term weight maintenance and to examine the strategies that were successful. An estimated 5,000 people participate in the NWCR. Participants may register if they have maintained at least a 30-pound weight loss for more than a year. After studying these individuals, Hill and his colleagues described the keys to their weight loss success in a 2005 article. In essence, no one plan or diet was common to all participants. Weight loss was maintained by a variety of personally designed diet and exercise strategies. Many participants had tried and failed several times before they were able to find the lifestyle and diet patterns that worked for them. Methods that were common to most participants were eating a relatively low-fat diet, eating breakfast, self-monitoring through food records, weighing themselves regularly, and regular physical activity (about one hour per day) (Hill et al. 2005).

At present, no strategies are defined that will help the majority of obese and overweight people successfully manage their weight given an environment that encourages overeating and less and less physical activity. Because millions of people are overweight or obese, they are a diverse group and will take many routes to success.

Medications

Nonprescription

Numerous over-the-counter (OTC) weight-loss products are available. Most have not been proven to be effective and safe. During the past decades, products for weight loss have had to change their formulations based on new government regulations and warnings. For example, amphetamines, originally developed as a treatment for narcolepsy, were introduced in 1937 as weight-loss drugs when they were found to reduce appetite as well as keep people awake. An amphetamine-type drug, desoxyephedrine, was approved by the FDA for obesity treatment in 1947. It warned against its use in persons with "cardiovascular disease, hypertension, or insomnia" and in those who were "neurotic or hyperexcitable" (Colman 2004).

In 1960, amphetamines were the most commonly prescribed medications for obesity (Parry et al. 1973). However, amphetamines were not without risks. Accelerated heart rate, increased blood pressure, hallucinations, psychiatric disorders, addiction, withdrawal problems, and heart failure were side effects that brought about the end of the amphetamine era. In the 1970s, government agencies all over the world placed tighter restrictions on drugs with the potential for abuse. Stimulant drugs are well established in treatment of obesity, and amphetamines are still approved for use under tight regulations in most countries.

Ephedra

Ephedra, also commonly known as Ma Huang, has been used in Chinese medicine for more than 2,500 years. It is made of dried branches of an evergreen shrub–like plant native to Central Asia and Mongolia. The principal active ingredient, ephedrine, is a compound that can powerfully stimulate the nervous system and heart. Ephedrine is chemically similar to amphetamines and may decrease appetite and increase metabolism. From the 1980s, ephedra had been popular for increasing energy and enhancing athletic performance, and it was used in many dietary supplements marketed for weight loss in the United States. It was a popular weight loss pill until it was banned in the United States by the FDA in 2004 because of safety concerns. In April 2005, a federal District Court judge in Utah overturned the ban in response to a suit brought by an ephedra manufacturer. The FDA appealed this lower court ruling, and in August 2006 the U.S. Court of Appeals for the Tenth Circuit upheld the FDA's original ban. With 19,000 adverse events reported, it was concluded that no dose of ephedrine was safe, and the sale of these products in the United States was made illegal. Up until this ruling, many supplement companies marketed low-dose ephedra products containing 10 milligrams (mg) or less of ephedra. According to the FDA, little evidence exists to show that ephedra is effective except for short-term weight loss. The increased risk of increased blood pressure, heart attacks, strokes, or seizures outweighs any benefits (NCCAM 2006).

Another drug, phenylpropanolamine, originally used to treat nasal congestion, also had the side effect of appetite suppression and was used in nonprescription diet aids for weight loss. One such product was Dexatrim—a popular appetite suppressant for more than 25 years. Phenylpropanolamine was Dexatrim's primary ingredient, but it was removed from the product line because of side effects such as increased risk for bleeding in the brain. Dexatrim switched its focus to ephedrine-based pills until ephedrine was banned by the FDA. After the ban, manufacturers of diet and weight-loss drugs like Dexatrim turned their attention to finding alternatives that would mimic its effects.

Dexatrim products are now drug free. They are based on a blend of guarana, kola nut, and bitter orange as well as several vitamins and minerals; green tea extract is also a common ingredient. They may or may not contain caffeine. Some side effects may include dizziness, nausea, high blood pressure, and depression. Dexatrim does point out that its diet aid works best when used with a sensible meal plan and regular exercise. It advertises that dieters will see results in one to two weeks when diet, exercise, and Dexatrim diet pills are combined. The truth is that most people could probably achieve the same results with diet and exercise alone.

The Metabolife line is another group of popular OTC products. Metabolife 356, an ephedra-based supplement, once generated hundreds of millions of dollars in annual sales. Metabolife 356, like other ephedra-containing supplements, was linked to thousands of serious adverse events, so it was discontinued following the FDA ban on ephedra-containing dietary supplements. Currently, Metabolife offers various supplements for weight-loss or weight-maintenance phases that may contain caffeine; vitamins; minerals; and caffeine-containing extracts of green tea, guarana, and yerba mate. Even without the effective ephedra, the plan still claims that the supplement will control appetite and burn fat. Metabolife also recommends that its products be combined with a healthy diet and exercise program. To support that advice, an online program helps customers plan and track weight-loss goals through education, tips from the experts, and community encouragement. The Web site features a collection of healthy recipes; suggestions for strength-training exercises; weight-management tips; and logs to track goals, diet, fitness, and results. Using Metabolife without changes in lifestyle will not be helpful for weight loss because it does not contain ingredients that have been proven to achieve effective results in the long run. The FDA does not support the weight-loss promises made by Metabolife.

For people who are wondering whether any OTC weight-loss medications work, the answer is, maybe. Although some ingredients like caffeine or tea that increase energy expenditure may be helpful for weight control, the concentration of these ingredients in diet preparations probably is too small to have an effect on weight loss in most people. A few cups of coffee or tea could have a similar outcome, taste better, and cost much less.

Herbs and Supplements

A popular question among people who are looking for more ways to control weight is, What herbs or supplements should I take to lose weight? A survey indicated that more than a quarter of American women trying to lose weight tried over-the-counter weight-loss supplements (Blanck, Khan, and Serdula 2001). The products promise a wide variety of ways to reduce fat, including increasing energy expenditure, increasing satiety, increasing fat oxidation, and blocking dietary fat and carbohydrate absorption. In terms of OTC weight-loss products, 64 percent of consumers think the government requires warnings about potential side effects, 54 percent believe these products are approved for safety by the FDA, and 46 percent think the products are approved for efficacy. In addition, 37 percent of consumers believe that herbal supplements are safer than prescription or OTC medications (Pillitteri et al. 2008). None of these beliefs is true. Although claims that dietary supplements can prevent, mitigate, treat, or cure a specific disease cannot be legally made, this distinction becomes clouded for many weight-loss products. Misleading weight-loss claims are seemingly everywhere, preying on consumers desperate for an easy solution. Current regulatory processes are weak, underfunded, and understaffed. This situation must be corrected and federal agencies must aggressively pursue manufacturers of those products that make unsubstantiated claims targeted toward vulnerable populations.

Supplements are attractive because they often advertise remarkable benefits and they are marketed as "natural," which may be interpreted as an assurance of safety and efficacy. The choice to supplement a diet with particular botanicals, vitamins, minerals, or other products can be a sensible decision that improves well-being and vitality. How do we sift through the false claims or junk science to find accurate information about supplements and their side effects or benefits? Because there is no official recommended dose for supplements, distributors are free to say whatever they want to about products. Intriguing research findings may be seen in animals; however, rats and mice are not people. Clinical trials with humans are necessary to know if the supplements are truly effective. Only carefully controlled scientific studies can show whether a product actually works. The best information is based on the results of rigorous scientific testing, rather than on testimonials or anecdotes. Some supplement suppliers accuse scientists of trying to keep secrets about alternative products that have miraculous powers. However, scientists are interested in studying the benefits and the risks of dietary supplements. The federal government even has an agency, the National Center for Complementary and Alternative Medicine (NCCAM), devoted to rigorous scientific research (http://www.nccam.nih.gov). Anyone can get information on thousands of studies from NCCAM.

Red Flag Campaign

The allure of a magic elixir can tempt anyone who wants an easy way to lose weight. Consumers spend roughly $1 billion a year on heavily advertised weight-loss products that are at best unproven and at worst unsafe. They promote unrealistic expectations and false hopes. In September 2002, the U.S. Federal Trade Commission (FTC) released a report titled *Weight Loss Advertising: An Analysis of Current Trends* indicating that the use of false and misleading claims in weight-loss advertising was widespread (FTC 2002). Researchers examined 300 weight-loss advertisements taken from television, radio, the Internet, newspapers, magazines, e-mail, and direct mail. The Commission found that 55 percent of weight-loss ads made claims that were misleading, lacked proof, or were obviously false. Although the FTC study did not criticize specific products, it provided numerous examples of false or exaggerated claims and said some weight-loss supplements lacked safety warnings and could be dangerous.

The FTC Division of Advertising Practices is responsible for enforcing federal truth-in-advertising laws. A major initiative was the 2003 Red Flag program, which encourages the media to screen out weight-loss advertisements that contain false claims. It also advises consumers to be wary of any product that claims fast and easy weight loss results. The following is a list of red flags that alert the public and the media that an advertising claim should be met with a healthy portion of skepticism.

Red flags are claims that a product can:

- Cause weight loss of 2 pounds or more a week for a month or more without dieting or exercise.
- Cause substantial weight loss no matter what or how much the consumer eats.
- Cause permanent weight loss (even when the consumer stops using the product).
- Block the absorption of fat or calories to enable consumers to lose substantial weight.
- Safely enable consumers to lose more than 3 pounds per week for more than four weeks.
- Cause substantial weight loss for all users.

- Produce weight-loss results that exceed what is physiologically possible under normal circumstances, as claimed by testimonials, for example, losing 120 pounds in seven weeks (FTC 2003).

Dietary Fiber

This food component has also been linked to weight regulation. A review summarizing the effects of high- versus low-fiber diet interventions found that the high-fiber diets increased satiety and decreased subsequent appetite. Because the average dietary fiber intake in the United States is approximately half the USDA recommendation of 25 to 30 grams per day, increasing dietary fiber may be a simple way to help decrease the prevalence of obesity (Howarth, Saltzman, and Roberts 2001).

Example of Research Study in Detail: Chitosan

Fiber supplements and "fat blockers" have been advertised as ways to prevent fat absorption. Following is an example of research that shows how scientists assessed the claims and effectiveness of chitosan, a fiber supplement, starting with some background on the product.

Chitosan is a calorie-free, high-fiber carbohydrate. It is produced commercially by chemically altering chitin, which is the structural element in the shells of crustaceans such as crabs, shrimp, and lobsters. As a food ingredient, chitosan adds thickness and a smooth texture to food products and is used in applications such as thickening chocolate milk drinks. Chitosan also has been approved by the FDA for use as an edible film to protect foods from dehydration. Like other forms of fiber, such as bran, chitosan is not well digested by the human body. Chitosan's configuration allows it to bind to fats and cholesterol. Its calorie-reducing effect is ascribed to its purported ability to bind with ingested fat and carry it out of the digestive tract. It has been used in Japan in several types of foods, including soybean paste, potato chips, and noodles, to help prevent fat absorption. A Japanese confection called Choco Lady is a sweet chocolate pellet that contains a crispy chitosan-enriched center. The pellets are claimed to help with weight loss. The product description states, "For maximum effect, the consumer is advised to eat five pellets before each meal . . . targeted towards men and women who tend to eat greasy meals" (*AFJ* 2006).

Apart from its role as a food additive, chitosan is sold as a dietary supplement with claims that it will block the absorption of significant amounts of dietary fat and lead to rapid weight loss. In support of the fat-blocking claim was a demonstration aired on the QVC television channel. A beaker was filled with oil and a water-based liquid to simulate what happens in a person's gastrointestinal tract, even though a beaker does not actually simulate human digestion. When the oil and water did not mix, chitosan was added to the concoction. The TV camera showed clumps of chitosan. This demonstration is offered as "proof" that chitosan combines with fat, prevents it from being absorbed by the body, and will lead to rapid weight loss. If chitosan were to work as claimed, an increased amount of fat would appear in the feces after a person consumes chitosan along with meals containing fat. A series of studies that measured the amount of fat in feces of a total of 104 men and women taking chitosan were published in 2005 (Gades and Stern 2005). These data were compared with data from a control period. Three different brands of chitosan were tested. The greatest amount of fat that was excreted in men was 1.8 grams per day, or 16 calories. At that rate, it would take more than 15 months to lose about 2 pounds of body fat using chitosan. It did not block the absorption of any fat in women. A systematic review of randomized controlled trials of chitosan indicated that the effect of chitosan on body weight was minimal and unlikely to be of clinical significance (Mhurchu et al. 2005).

Prescription Drugs

All drugs have side effects, some of which are serious. Drugs for chronic diseases are taken for long periods of time. For example, if a person has high blood pressure, takes a drug to treat the disease, and subsequently stops taking the drug, blood pressure increases. The FDA has different standards for approval of drugs for treating obesity: (1) The FDA requires that obesity drugs have been tested clinically for at least a year. (2) No side effects should be present. (3) The drug is only prescribed for a limited time—usually a few months.

When considering weight-loss prescription medication, it is assumed that when a patient stops taking a drug, the patient will not regain lost weight. At this time, drug therapy and life style interventions are not opposing strategies; the current drugs used for weight loss are combined with lifestyle interventions.

Fen-Phen

In 1992, a University of Rochester professor first promoted the drug combination of fenfluramine and phentermine, or fen-phen, as a magic weight-loss pill. Studies had shown that the combination could be used in lower dosages with fewer side effects than either drug alone (e.g., Weintraub et al. 1984). Participants of a four-year research project lost an average of about 31 pounds on fen-phen, versus about 10 pounds on a placebo (see Glossary for the definition of "placebo"), after 34 weeks and were able to keep the weight off over the long term (Weintraub et al. 1992). Although the initial rationale for the combination was that the two drugs would provide an additive action, allowing the use of lower, safer doses of each drug, reviewers from Texas A&M University concluded that the combination was not merely additive but also synergistic—that is, they were more effective together than simply doubling the dose of either drug alone. Mass marketing of this combination of drugs took place, and the number of prescriptions written for fen-phen grew from 60,000 in 1992 to 18 million in 1996 (Langreth 1997). Hundreds of clinics opened specifically to prescribe these weight-loss medications. It seemed as though researchers had finally found the magic pill for weight loss and long-term weight control.

The drug was extensively used until a report from the Mayo Clinic linked 24 cases of heart valve disease, which included severe deformity and leakage, to use of the medications. These 24 cases, all women, had no previous history of cardiovascular disease. The leakage was caused by a buildup of abnormal tissue on the valves of their heart that prevented them from sealing properly. This type of valve damage is a silent condition, causing no symptoms until it becomes severe, is life threatening, and requires surgery to repair. Another investigation showed that 271 of 291 patients who had taken fen-phen showed abnormal electrocardiograms. In 1997, American Home Products, fen-phen's manufacturer, removed the drug from the market (Langreth 1997). The 50-year-old generic drug phentermine, which was one half of the fen-phen combination, does not show these serious side effects and is still on the market.

Meridia

The FDA has since approved a long-term appetite suppressant, Meridia. Meridia is the brand name for sibutramine, a selective serotonin reuptake inhibitor, or SSRI. The drug prevents recycling (re-uptake) of noradrenaline and serotonin. Noradrenaline and serotonin are neurotransmitters that enhance the feeling of satisfaction from eating. Weight loss with sibutramine is increased when positive changes are made in diet and lifestyle. In one trial, people with an initial BMI of 30–40 who had lost weight when given sibutramine for four weeks continued to lose weight during 44 additional weeks of sibutramine treatment. In this study, people were simply told to eat a healthy diet. However, in a more recent study, a much higher amount of weight loss was achieved when sibutramine treatment was combined with lifestyle-modification counseling. Those who had sibutramine alone lost an average of 11 pounds after a year, while those in the sibutramine and counseling group had an average weight loss of 26 pounds (Rubio et al. 2007).

The neurotransmitters that control appetite also control numerous other body processes, so side effects from sibutramine are common. The drug is not recommended for people with hypertension because it increases blood pressure in some individuals. Other reported side effects include constipation, dry mouth, headache, and increased heart rate. Meridia also has been associated with more serious problems. Between February 1998 and September 2001, hundreds of people throughout the world who took Meridia were hospitalized, and the FDA reported that 29 people taking Meridia in the United States had died (Wolfe, Sasich, and Barbenhenn 2002).

Sibutramine has also encountered regulatory problems. Warnings about its safety have been issued in France and the United Kingdom. In 2002, the Italian Ministry of Health suspended sales of the drug after 50 reports of adverse events and two deaths. However, the European Union Committee for Proprietary Medicinal Products later issued a report stating that, when used according to directions, sibutramine had a favorable risk/benefit ratio. The manufacturer, Abbott Laboratories, had reported that the death rate among patients taking the drug (12,000 people in clinical trials and 8.5 million patients worldwide) was substantially lower than what would normally occur in any obese patient population (Abbott Laboratories 2002).

In 2002, the FDA conducted an investigation into the safety of the drug. The present protocol for sibutramine, issued as a result of the investigation, indicates that it should be used only by people who are at least 30 pounds overweight who do not have cardiovascular problems.

Orlistat

Hoffmann–La Roche's Xenical is the brand name for orlistat, an obesity drug that can be taken for an extended time period. It blocks fat-digesting enzymes in the intestine called lipases and prevents some dietary fat from being digested and absorbed. It is usually taken three times a day, before main meals that contain fat. Up to 30 percent absorption of dietary fat can be blocked with 120 mg of orlistat taken with a meal. This extra fat that passes down the intestine may cause abdominal pain, gas, oily stools, and fecal incontinence, especially if the fat content of the meal is high. This effect persuades users to limit their fat intake.

A meta-analysis of Xenical trials showed that the drug helped dieting patients lose an average of 2 to 3 percent of their body weight compared with dieting alone. After one year of treatment, about one-third more patients treated with orlistat three times per day lost a greater percentage of body weight than those treated with placebo. In a number of studies, orlistat treatment significantly improved blood pressure, lowered levels of LDL cholesterol (bad cholesterol) in the blood, and lowered fasting blood glucose and insulin levels. Results from a four-year study suggested that development of type 2 diabetes, especially in those with impaired glucose tolerance, was delayed with orlistat use (Heymsfield et al. 2000). The majority of subjects across the studies gained the weight back after discontinuing the drug.

Orlistat has been approved for over-the-counter sales as the product Alli. It contains about half the dose of the prescription drug. The package insert cautions that, while the product does prevent fat absorption, it may cause oily bowel movements so frequently that it suggests consumers wear a panty liner when starting the treatment.

Rimonabant

The brand name for rimonabant is Acomplia (Zimulti in Europe) and is marketed by Sanofi-Aventis. It acts, both in the brain and in other parts of the body, to increase feelings of fullness, and it plays a role in the metabolism of glucose and fat in the body.

Rimonabant is an inhibitor of cannabinoid type 1 receptors, which are widely distributed in the brain and in other tissues, including on fat cells. Interestingly, these receptors affect intake of sweet or fatty foods. These same receptors are also involved in nicotine addiction; thus, rimonabant is also prescribed to help people quit smoking. Overeaters and smokers have been shown to have very active cannabinoid type 1 receptors. Rimonabant is usually taken as a single dose before breakfast. In clinical trials in people with BMI values of 34–38 who took rimonabant, participants taking rimonabant had a significantly greater weight loss after one year compared with those given a placebo. By continuing rimonabant treatment for a second year, weight loss was maintained. Subjects who were switched to a placebo regained most of the weight they had lost in the first year (Rubio et al. 2007). Acomplia was introduced in Europe in 2006 and is also available in several other countries. Sanofi-Aventis withdrew its application to market Acomplia in the United States after an FDA advisory panel unanimously recommended against approving the drug because of its side effects, including risk of depression and suicide.

Response to drug therapy varies among individuals, and no one drug works for all people. Diet drugs will not force anyone to stop eating, as most people eat in response to environmental cues rather than physiologic hunger. Medical professionals are beginning to understand that regain of weight upon stopping medication is not treatment failure, but rather it indicates that obesity is a chronic disease much like diabetes. Drugs are not a quick fix for a disease that requires long-term treatment. As risks are inherent in taking any medication, research is needed to assess the long-term safety of obesity drugs relative to the health risks of obesity and overweight. Since obesity is a chronic disease, it would be helpful to have weight loss medications that can be used for long periods of time, such as those used for treatmentment of hypertension and dyslipidemia.

Obesity (Bariatric) Surgery

In 1954, Dr. Arnold Kremen and Dr. John Linner at the University of Minnesota were studying nutrition absorption in dogs. They discovered that the dogs lost weight after they underwent operations that bypassed much of their intestines (Kremen, Linner, and Nelson 1954). After Dr. Linner went into private surgical practice, one of his patients asked him to use the technique on her in the hope that she, too, could lose weight. With the successful results of that procedure, bariatric surgery was born. In 1991, a National Institutes of Health (NIH) expert panel endorsed bypass surgery for obesity when they reviewed what was known about surgical treatments for severely overweight individuals. It concluded that surgical alterations of the digestive system appeared to work for many people without severe side effects. It approved bariatric surgery as an effective option for severely obese people who have failed more moderate weight-reduction strategies. In 1999, singer Carnie Wilson had gastric bypass surgery and allowed the procedure to be broadcast live over the Internet. The broadcast was viewed by more than 500,000 people. Sixteen months after the procedure, Carnie had lost 152 pounds of her original weight of more than 300 pounds. She was a celebrated example of successful weight-loss surgery and even posed for *Playboy Magazine* in 2003. In 2005, after she gave birth to her daughter, the pounds began to come back. In 2008, she weighed more than 200 pounds—her weight increased but still down about 100 pounds from her heaviest. That the weight may be eventually regained demonstrates a limitation of obesity surgery. On the other hand, an important health benefit is that the procedure may allow individuals to gain many years of reduced risk related to high levels of obesity.

Official guidelines consider weight-loss surgery appropriate for adults with severe obesity (BMI ≥ 40, or 37–39.9 if accompanied by other conditions such as diabetes) who have not reached a satisfactory weight through diet, exercise, and medication. Surgery may be used as the initial treatment if BMI is greater than or equal to 50. It is major surgery, undertaken only by specialist hospital teams, and is not without risks. People who have weight-loss surgery will need continuing specialist medical support for many years. Weight-loss surgery is not advised in children, except in extreme circumstances.

Three main types of weight-loss surgery are currently used: gastric banding, gastric bypass, and duodenal switch/biliopancreatic diversion. In gastric banding, a small pouch is made in the upper part of the stomach with an adjustable band. During eating, this smaller pouch fills up quickly, produces a sensation of fullness, and reduces food intake. The food passes slowly into the main part of the stomach and then on to the rest of the digestive system. A remarkable feature of the gastric band is that it can be adjusted without additional surgery. The band is actually a balloon filled with saline solution that can be inflated or deflated. This operation causes weight loss by reducing food intake, leaves the main part of the digestive system unchanged, and is easily reversible. It typically produces a 40 to 50 percent loss of excess body weight in the two years after surgery (WIN 2008).

During the gastric bypass procedure, the top section of the stomach is partitioned to make a new mini-stomach. This pouch is connected to a lower section of the small intestine, bypassing the upper part where most active digestion takes place. Food does not get normal breakdown in the smaller stomach, and absorption of nutrients from the small intestine is greatly reduced. Weight loss is caused by both restriction and reduced absorption of food. The surgery results in about 55 to 65 percent of excess body weight. In a duodenal switch, the stomach pouch is reduced in size and left connected to the upper small intestine, which is then shortened. Similar to gastric bypass, weight loss occurs with the combination of reduced food intake and reduced absorption, and 65 to 75 percent of excess weight is typically lost (WIN 2008).

The surgeries can either be performed via laparoscopic surgery (two small incisions in the abdominal wall) or via open surgery (one larger incision in the abdominal wall). How is the decision made as to which surgical procedure to use? A number of studies report death rates in people who received bariatric surgery. Usually, a lower complication rate is associated with laparoscopic surgery. However, for very obese patients, with a BMI of greater than 80, laparoscopic surgery is not done. At this time, a large enough database of obesity surgery results, including benefits and complications, is not available for individual patients to be able to assess the risk for a given type of bariatric surgery (Wolfe and Morton 2005). For people with cardiovascular disease (CVD), a national database houses data for individuals that includes blood values that are risk indicators such as cholesterol or triglycerides, physical symptoms, and the outcomes of various treatments (NCEP 2001). For patients with CVD, a physician may present the options to the patient and, weighing the benefits and risks, potentially choose the "best" treatment for an individual. At this time, this approach is not possible for obese patients. In terms of outcomes for obese patients who are candidates for bariatric surgery, the construction of a database has begun, but it may be as long as 10 years before it is fully functional.

Obesity Surgery Cautions and Controversies

Pros

Most patients experience rapid weight loss and continue to do so for 12 to 18 months following obesity surgery. Patients may maintain 50 to 60 percent of their weight loss 10 to 14 years after obesity surgery. Strong evidence exists to show that obesity surgery works in older adults. For example, when patients older than 65 years are only treated medically for severe obesity, the prevalence of comorbidities increases after a year. In contrast, surgically treated older patients experience a decrease in the prevalence of comorbidities (Miller and Kral 2008). NIH guidelines for bariatric surgery do not provide any age criteria (NIH 1992).

Cons

Several risks are associated with obesity surgery, including a 10 percent or higher risk of complications. Ten to 20 percent of patients needed follow-up operations to correct obesity surgery complications such as abdominal hernias. Gallstones develop in more than one-third of patients. Anemia, osteoporosis, and other bone diseases are the result of nutritional deficiencies that develop after the obesity surgery. The possible death rate is 1 out of 200 cases. This rate is lower for more experienced surgeons who perform at least 150 operations yearly (Morino et al. 2007). Blue Cross and Blue Shield of North Carolina's assessment of results of surgery for morbid obesity showed that success rates were highly variable in their coverage area. Some surgeons had significant complication rates of 25 to 50 percent. By reviewing the claims data, the company found that patients of physicians who performed bariatric procedures more often had lower complication rates. Complications included such events as gastrointestinal tract leakage, bowel obstruction, bleeding, infections, complications from anesthesia, and death. With the expectation that the complication rate should be less than 10 percent during the first 60 days, Blue Cross identified those programs that consistently delivered high-quality results as Bariatric Surgery Centers of Excellence (BCBSNC 2008).

Despite much progress in developing safer and more effective surgical techniques, obesity surgery remains a last option for patients attempting weight loss. In addition, surgical candidates must be willing to radically change the way they eat to reflect the very much smaller amount of food (and water) that can be consumed at one time. One of the side effects of this surgery is the decreased absorption of some vitamins. Patients take a prescribed multivitamin pill that has larger doses of vitamins than the standard multivitamin supplement. People who have Guillain-Barré syndrome may not achieve an ideal body weight or a normal BMI range. The surgery commonly allows patients to reduce 50 percent of their *excess* weight. A person who is 100 pounds overweight could theoretically maintain a 50-pound loss and be healthier but still overweight. Long-term weight loss is not effortless after bariatric surgery. Lifestyle change is still necessary. For many people, the stomach pouch enlarges, intestinal absorption increases, and weight can be regained if diet and physical activity are not changed also.

Other Invasive Treatments for Obesity

Jaw Wiring

In 1977, the concept of wiring the jaws together was introduced. Jaw wiring can be performed in a dentist's chair. It is a painless procedure that takes less than an hour to perform. This orthodontic method of weight control prevents consumption of solid food, thus causing a reduction in calorie intake. Once the desired weight loss is achieved, the wiring is removed. The success rate of jaw wiring as a long-term method of achieving a normal weight is very low. Most patients do not discover a new, healthful way of eating; in fact, some are able to sip enough high-calorie fluids through a straw that no weight is lost. Large clinical studies demonstrated a median weight loss of 55 pounds with jaw wiring, but after four months the weight loss reached a plateau. When the wires were removed, patients regained 100 percent of the lost weight (Farquhar et al. 1986).

Liposuction

Liposuction is the most popular form of cosmetic surgery. It is a surgical procedure that removes fat deposits from areas under the skin (abdomen, thighs, buttocks, neck, back of arms) that do not respond to traditional weight-loss methods. The fat is extracted with a vacuum-suction canula (a hollow pen-like instrument) or with an ultrasonic probe that breaks up the fat and then removes it with suction. The cosmetic effect of liposuction may be very good, and many patients report being satisfied.

Liposuction is not a cure for obesity, because relatively little body fat (less than 10 pounds) can be removed safely. Some side effects include unusual lumpiness or dents in the skin, excessive bleeding, and negative response to general or local anesthesia. Because fat removal is considered a cosmetic procedure, most medical insurance will not pay for liposuction. The fat that is removed may come back with weight gain. Furthermore, the fat may appear in areas of the body where it did not previously occur (CDRH 2002).

How Does the Health Care System Deal with Obesity?

The health care system has a responsibility to play an active role in the management of obesity, and physicians are a first line of defense in addressing the issue. A major barrier to successful weight management is the lack of communication between patients and their health care providers. Despite the current focus on obesity and health care risks, less than half of obese patients are advised by their physicians to lose weight. Seventy-five percent of patients surveyed indicated that they looked to their physician a "slight amount" or "not at all" for help with weight control (Wadden and Foster 2000). When physicians mention weight, they often do not give useful, actionable information. Because patients have trouble losing weight and maintaining weight loss, they need ongoing support and reinforcement from health care providers. According to Dr. William Dietz:

> The kind of care delivery system necessary for chronic diseases like obesity is different from the traditional patient-provider relationship. So many patients in the United States are overweight that the one-to-one provider-patient relationship is probably archaic. It is based on an acute care model whereby the U.S. medical system has evolved to treat infectious diseases or injuries. It did not evolve to treat chronic diseases, and it did not evolve around prevention. Providers are not financially rewarded when they prevent disease; they are rewarded when patients get sick or need hospitalization (Pellerin 2005).

Opinion varies widely about how health care providers should manage obesity in the medical office or clinic. Physicians are often reluctant to discuss weight-related issues with patients. Such discussions are time consuming, and no solutions are available that apply to everyone. Several studies have shown that physician advice encouraging weight management significantly increases patients' attempts to lose weight (e.g., Loureiro and Nayga 2006). Experts recommend that doctors weigh and measure all their adult patients and refer obese ones to intensive counseling and behavioral treatment. An individual may want to lose weight but not be ready to make a focused commitment. Health care providers can assess patient willingness to change and educate patients about the effects of overweight on health by discussing results of physical exams, lab tests, and family history. Reduction of excess weight requires concentration and sustained effort. In cases where family- or work-related stress interferes with that effort, the treatment goal may simply be prevention of further weight gain (Wadden and Foster 2000).

All patients, no matter their weight, can benefit from lifestyle guidance to prevent weight gain. This advice and education will become part of good health care if insurance companies reimburse for obesity management as they do for control and prevention of diabetes. To deal with the obesity issue, Kaiser Permanente, a leading health maintenance organization in the United States, has adopted some of these recommendations for adults. One policy requires that all adult patients be evaluated for obesity. Those who are obese or at risk of becoming obese should be offered appropriate long-term interventions, as suggested by the NHLBI guidelines shown in Figure 6.2 in Chapter 6. The algorithm in Figure 6.2 depicts the NHLBI Expert Panel's treatment decision process, which provides a step-by-step approach to managing overweight and obese patients.

Interventions may include individual or group behavior change therapy, pharmaceutical intervention, or surgery for those at highest risk. A crucial step is to provide a variety of programs that can actually help patients manage weight. Because there is no single approach that works for everyone, the most effective interventions offer a number of programs that apply to specific groups. Overall, the most successful strategies rely on an active lifestyle that includes reasonable amounts of healthful foods. While pursuing these health strategies individuals may need to explore personal associations between emotions and eating habits. Programs may use Web-based resources alone or combined with conventional lifestyle management classes or one-on-one sessions.

With support from health care professionals, self-management is a cornerstone of therapy. Providers cannot be expected to manage weight for their patients. There are no guarantees for any medical treatment, including surgery, for long-term weight loss. The role of the provider is to help patients identify and solve problems that make it difficult for them to maintain a healthy weight. In the end, using the resources currently available, patients must make the choices and manage their problems for themselves.

Why Can't We Just Prevent Obesity?

Prevention has the potential to help decrease obesity, but no studies have been conducted for a long enough period to indicate what method(s) of prevention will work. Health care professionals and patients continue to question whether they can afford to wait for better evidence. Should we keep trying the methods we now have, and hope that they work for some people? The experts' best guesses, given current knowledge, are to encourage people to be more active; reduce marketing of unhealthful foods; and make foods like fruits and vegetables more affordable, attractive, and easily available.

The individual, the family, schools, workplaces, local and state government, and communities and organizations have to be part of the solution. To help people choose healthful foods, government agencies can require that food companies, restaurants, and caterers provide information about the calorie content of foods on menus and menu boards. To help people become more active, walking and bike riding should be encouraged; people may substitute bike riding and walking for going to a movie or watching television. To help prevent obesity in children, families can focus on being active together. On a community level, this means construction of safe bike lanes and paths. At work, walking stairs can be made more attractive than taking elevators. Also helpful is making people aware of healthy choices. In one study conducted at a railroad station in the Philadelphia, Pennsylvania, business district, more commuters chose the stairs over the escalator when a cartoon was visible showing a healthy heart walking the stairs and a sick-looking heart taking the escalator (Dolan et al. 2006).

A potentially successful model for obesity prevention would encompass dietary, activity, behavioral, pharmacological, and surgical components geared toward individual needs. To resolve the questions and controversies surrounding obesity, we need more scientifically based research into lifestyle or medical approaches that will make it easier for anyone to maintain a healthful energy balance. People in the United States depend upon the NIH to increase our understanding of the forces that contribute to obesity and to develop strategies for obesity prevention and treatment. The 27 institutes and centers of NIH provide direction and financial support through competitive grants to researchers in the United States and throughout the world. Currently, the NIH funds more than 90 percent of all obesity research in the United States. It is critically important to increase funding for obesity research in public and private sectors. The choice is ours: We can either learn more about how to effectively prevent obesity or spend billions and billions of dollars treating people with obesity.

Conclusions

No one can escape the basic law of nature that governs weight gain or loss—any energy consumed as food and not used through activity must be stored in the body as fat. However, people vary in their eating and exercise habits; in their genetic susceptibility to gaining weight; and in their individual metabolic rate, which determine weight gain or loss. Scientists have discovered a great deal about how weight gain occurs and some methods that may be effective in reversing it, although there is still much to learn. Inability to lose excess weight often has more to do with social, psychological, and behavioral factors than with metabolism. Both physiology and society work against people's weight-loss attempts. The automatic slowdown in our metabolic rate with weight loss, an evolutionary protection to prevent starvation, works against us when we try to lose excess weight. Influences of food advertising and the customs of social eating add to the difficulty. In short, weight management is not easy for most people.

References

Abbott Laboratories. "Meridia Safety." 2002. [Online information; retrieved 1/6/09.] http://www.meridia-rx.com/diet-pills/meridia/meridia_safety.htm.

Asian Food Journal (AFJ). "Choco Lady (Japan)." 2006. [Online information; retrieved 1/6/09.] http://www.asiafoodjournal.com/print.asp?id=3580.

Atkinson, R. L., N. V. Dhurandhar, D. B. Allison, R. L. Bowen, B. A. Israel, J. B. Albu, and A. S. Augustus. "Human Adenovirus-36 Is Associated with Increased Body Weight and Paradoxical Reduction of Serum Lipids." *International Journal of Obesity (London)* 29, no. 3 (2005): 281–286.

Ayyad, C., and T. Andersen. "Long-term Efficacy of Dietary Treatment of Obesity: A Systematic Review of Studies Published Between 1931 and 1999." *Obesity Reviews* 1, no. 2 (2000): 113–119.

Bellisle, F., and A. Drewnowski. "Intense Sweeteners, Energy Intake and the Control of Body Weight." *European Journal of Clinical Nutrition* 61 (2007): 691–700.

Bish, C. L., H. M. Blanck, M. K. Serdula, M. Marcus, H. W. Kohl III, and L. K. Khan. "Diet and Physical Activity Behaviors among Americans Trying to Lose Weight: 2000 Behavioral Risk Factor Surveillance System." *Obesity Research* 13, no. 3 (2005): 596–607.

Blanck, H. M., L. K. Khan, and M. K. Serdula. "Use of Nonprescription Weight Loss Products: Results from a Multistate Survey." *Journal of the American Medical Association* 286, no. 8 (2001): 930–935.

Blue Cross and Blue Shield of North Carolina (BCBSNC). "Bariatric Surgery Centers—Frequently asked questions." 2008. [Online information; retrieved 1/6/09.] http://www.bcbsnc.com/apps/coe/public/bariatric.action?zipCode=null.

Bravata, D. M., L. Sanders, J. Huang, H. M. Krumholz, I. Olkin, C. D. Gardner, and D. M. Bravata. "Efficacy and Safety of Low-Carbohydrate Diets: A Systematic Review." *Journal of the American Medical Association* 289, no. 14 (2003): 1837–1850.

Bray, G. A., and C. M. Champagne. "Beyond Energy Balance: There Is More to Obesity than Kilocalories." *Journal of the American Dietetic Association* 105, no. 5, Suppl. 1 (2005): S17–S23.

Bray G. A., S. Paeratakul, and B. M. Popkin. Dietary Fat and Obesity: a Review of Animal, Clinical and Epidemiological Studies. *Physiology and Behavior* 83, no. 4 (2004): 549–555.

Carmona, R. "The Obesity Crisis in America." In *Testimony before the Subcommittee on Education Reform Committee on Education and the Workforce United States House of Representatives*, edited by Surgeon General, U.S. Public Health Service. Washington, DC: U.S. Department of Health and Human Services, 2003.

Center for Consumer Freedom (CFF). "Epidemic of Obesity Myths." Washington, DC: Center for Consumer Freedom, 2004.

Center for Devices and Radiological Health (CDRH). "Liposuction Information." Rockville, MD: U.S. Food and Drug Administration, 2002.

Center for Nutrition Policy and Promotion (CNPP). "MyPyramid Tracker." 2008. [Online information; retrieved 1/6/09.] http://www.mypyramidtracker.gov/.

Centers for Disease Control and Prevention (CDC). "U.S. Obesity Trends 1985–2006." Atlanta: CDC, 2007.

Christakis, N. A., and J. H. Fowler. "The Spread of Obesity in a Large Social Network over 32 Years." *New England Journal of Medicine* 357, no. 4 (2007): 370–379.

Colman, Eric. "FDA Regulation of Obesity Drugs: 1938–1999." 2004. [Online information; retrieved 1/6/09.] http://209.85.173.104/search?q=cache:jl2bdha0NM0J:www.fda.gov/ohrms/dockets/AC/04/slides/2004-4068S1_01_Colman.ppt+FDA+amphetamine+weight+loss&hl=en&ct=clnk&cd=1&gl=us.

Dhurandhar, N. V., B. A. Israel, J. M. Kolesar, G. F. Mayhew, M. E. Cook, and R. L. Atkinson. "Increased Adiposity in Animals Due to a Human Virus." *International Journal of Obesity-Related Metabolic Disorders* 24, no. 8 (2000): 989–996.

Dolan, M. S., L. A. Weiss, R. A. Lewis, A. Pietrobelli, M. Heo, and M. S. Faith. " 'Take the Stairs Instead of the Escalator': Effect of Environmental Prompts on Community Stair Use and Implications for a National 'Small Steps' Campaign." *Obesity Reviews* 7, no. 1 (2006): 25–32.

Ernsberger, P. "Obesity Is Hazardous to Your Health." *Debates in Medicine* 2 (1989): 102–137.

Farquhar, D. L., J. M. Griffiths, J. F. Munro, and F. Stevenson. "Unexpected Weight Regain Following Successful Jaw Wiring." *Scottish Medical Journal* 31, no. 3 (1986): 180.

Flegal, K. M., B. I. Graubard, D. F. Williamson, and M. H. Gail. "Excess Deaths Associated with Underweight, Overweight, and Obesity." *Journal of the American Medical Association* 293, no. 15 (2005): 1861–1867.

Foster, G. D., T. A. Wadden, S. Phelan, D. B. Sarwer, and R. S. Sanderson. "Obese Patients' Perceptions of Treatment Outcomes and the Factors that Influence Them." *Archives of Internal Medicine* 161, no. 17 (2001): 2133–2139.

Fujioka, K. "Management of Obesity as a Chronic Disease: Nonpharmacologic, Pharmacologic, and Surgical Options." *Obesity Research* 10, Suppl. 2 (2002): 116S–123S.

Gades, M. D., and J. S. Stern. "Chitosan Supplementation and Fat Absorption in Men and Women." *Journal of the American Dietetic Association* 105, no. 1 (2005): 72–77.

Gregg, E. W., Y. J. Cheng, B. L. Cadwell, G. Imperatore, D. E. Williams, K. M. Flegal, K. M. Narayan, and D. F. Williamson. "Secular Trends in Cardiovascular Disease Risk Factors According to Body Mass Index in US Adults." *Journal of the American Medical Association* 293, no. 15 (2005): 1868–1874.

Heymsfield, S. B., K. R. Segal, J. Hauptman, C. P. Lucas, M. N. Boldrin, A. Rissanen, J. P. Wilding, and L. Sjostrom. "Effects of Weight Loss with Orlistat on Glucose Tolerance and Progression to Type 2 Diabetes in Obese Adults." *Archives of Internal Medicine* 160, no. 9 (2000): 1321–1326.

Hill, J. O., H. Wyatt, S. Phelan, and R. Wing. "The National Weight Control Registry: Is It Useful in Helping Deal with Our Obesity Epidemic?" *Journal of Nutrition Education and Behavior* 37, no. 4 (2005): 206–210.

Howarth, N. C., E. Saltzman, and S. B. Roberts. "Dietary Fiber and Weight Regulation." *Nutrition Reviews* 59, no. 5 (2001): 129–139.

Hunt, R., N. L. Zorich, and A. B. Thomson. "Overview of Olestra: A New Fat Substitute." *Canadian Journal of Gastroenterology* 12, no. 3 (1998): 193–197.

Internal Revenue Service (IRS). "Internal Revenue Service Ruling 2002-19." Washington, DC: IRS, 2002.

Kazaks, A., and J. S. Stern. "Strategies to Reduce Calories in Foods." In *Handbook of Obesity, Clinical Applications*, edited by G. A. Bray and C. Bouchard, 417–424. New York: Informa Healthcare USA, 2008.

Kolakowski, Nick. "The Obesity Virus?" *DOC News*, January 1, 2005.

Kramer, F. M., R. W. Jeffery, J. L. Forster, and M. K. Snell. "Long-term Follow-up of Behavioral Treatment for Obesity: Patterns of Weight Regain among Men and Women." *International Journal of Obesity* 13, no. 2 (1989): 123–136.

Kremen, A. J., J. H. Linner, and C. H. Nelson. "An Experimental Evaluation of the Nutritional Importance of Proximal and Distal Small Intestine." *Annals of Surgery* 140, no. 3 (1954): 439–448.

Kretsch, M. J., A. K. Fong, and M. W. Green. "Behavioral and Body Size Correlates of Energy Intake Underreporting by Obese and Normal-Weight Women." *Journal of the American Dietetic Association* 99, no. 3 (1999): 300–306; quiz 307–308.

Langreth, R. "Critics Claim Diet Clinics Misuse Obesity Drugs." *Wall Street Journal*, March 31, 1997.

Levi, J., L. M. Segal, and E. Gadola. "F as in Fat: How Obesity Policies Are Failing in America—2007." Washington, DC: Trust for America's Health, 2007.

Loureiro, M. L., and R. M. Nayga Jr. "Obesity, Weight Loss, and Physician's Advice." *Social Science & Med* 62, no. 10 (2006): 2458–2468.

Mallone, C., and J. Bland-Campbell. "New Insights on the Away-From-Home Eating Patterns and Nutritional Preferences of Americans." 2005. [Online information; retrieved 1/29/09.] http://www.aramark.com/CaseStudyWhitePaperDetail.aspx?PostingID=420& ChannelID=221.

Mhurchu, C. N., C. Dunshea-Mooij, D. Bennett, and A. Rodgers. "Effect of Chitosan on Weight Loss in Overweight and Obese Individuals: A Systematic Review of Randomized Controlled Trials." *Obesity Reviews* 6, no. 1 (2005): 35–42.

Miller, M. E., and J. G. Kral. "Surgery for Obesity in Older Women." *Menopause International* 14, no. 4 (2008):155–162.

Morino, M., M. Toppino, P. Forestieri, L. Angrisani, M. E. Allaix, and N. Scopinaro. "Mortality after Bariatric Surgery: Analysis of 13,871 Morbidly Obese Patients from a National Registry." *Annals of Surgery* 246, no. 6 (2007): 1002–1007; discussion 1007–1009.

National Center for Complementary and Alternative Medicine (NCCAM). "Ephedra at a Glance." 2006. [Online information; retrieved 7/9/07.] http://nccam.nih.gov/health/ephedra/ataglance.htm.

National Center for Health Statistics (NCHS). Health, United States, 2007. With Chartbook on Trends in the Health of Americans. Vol (PHS) 2007-1232: Government Printing Office; 2007. http://www.cdc.gov/nchs/data/hus/hus07.pdf.

National Cholesterol Education Program (NCEP). "Executive Summary of the Third Report of the National Cholesterol Education Program (NCEP) Expert Panel on Detection, Evaluation, and Treatment of High Blood Cholesterol in Adults (Adult Treatment

Panel III)." *Journal of the American Medical Association* 285, no. 19 (2001): 2486–2497.

National Heart, Lung and Blood Institute (NHLBI). *Clinical Guidelines on the Identification, Evaluation, and Treatment of Overweight and Obesity in Adults: The Evidence Report.* Bethesda, MD: National Heart, Lung and Blood Institute, 1998.

National Institutes of Health (NIH). "Gastrointestinal Surgery for Severe Obesity: NIH Consensus Development Conference." *American Journal of Clinical Nutrition* 55, Suppl. 2 (1992): 615S–619S.

Parry, H. J., M. B. Balter, G. D. Mellinger, I. H. Cisin, and D. I. Manheimer. "National Patterns of Psychotherapeutic Drug Use." *Archives of General Psychiatry* 28, no. 6 (1973): 18–74.

Pellerin, C. "The Global Epidemic of Obesity." 2005. [Online information; retrieved 12/15/07.] http://usa.usembassy.de/etexts/sport/ijge0105.pdf.

Pillitteri, J. L., S. Shiffman, J. M. Rohay, A. M. Harkins, S. L. Burton, and T. A. Wadden. "Use of Dietary Supplements for Weight Loss in the United States: Results of a National Survey." *Obesity (Silver Spring)* 16, no. 4 (2008): 790–796.

Rubio, M. A., M. Gargallo, A. Isabel Millan, and B. Moreno. "Drugs in the Treatment of Obesity: Sibutramine, Orlistat and Rimonabant." *Public Health Nutrition* 10, no. 10A (2007): 1200–1205.

Stagg-Elliott, V. "Is Obesity a Disease? Clinicians Disagree." 2006. [Online information; retrieved 1/6/09.] http://www.ama-assn.org/amednews/2006/02/06/hlsa0206.htm.

Thomson, A. B., R. H. Hunt, and N. L. Zorich. "Review Article: Olestra and Its Gastrointestinal Safety." *Alimentary Pharmacology & Therapeutics* 12, no. 12 (1998): 1185–1200.

Tsai, A. G., and T. A. Wadden. "Systematic Review: An Evaluation of Major Commercial Weight Loss Programs in the United States." *Annals of Internal Medicine* 142, no. 1 (2005): 56–66.

U.S. Department of Health and Human Services (HHS). "HHS Announces Revised Medicare Obesity Coverage Policy." 2004. [Online news release; retrieved 1/6/09.] http://www.hhs.gov/news/press/2004pres/20040715.html.

U.S. Federal Trade Commission (FTC). "Red Flag: Bogus Weight Loss Claims." 2002. [Online information; retrieved 1/6/09.] http://www.ftc.gov/bcp/conline/edcams/redflag/falseclaims.html.

U.S. Federal Trade Commission (FTC). "Weight-Loss Advertising: An Analysis of Current Trends." Washington, DC: FTC, 2003.

Wadden, T. A., and G. D. Foster. "Behavioral Treatment of Obesity." *Medical Clinics of North America* 84, no. 2 (2000): 441–461, vii.

Wadden, T. A., J. A. Sternberg, K. A. Letizia, A. J. Stunkard, and G. D. Foster. "Treatment of Obesity by Very Low Calorie Diet, Behavior Therapy, and Their Combination: A Five-Year Perspective." *International Journal of Obesity* 13, Suppl. 2 (1989): 39–46.

Weight-control Information Network (WIN). "Bariatric Surgery for Severe Obesity." Bethesda, MD: National Institutes of Health, 2008.

Weintraub, M., J. D. Hasday, A. I. Mushlin, and D. H. Lockwood. "A Double-Blind Clinical Trial in Weight Control. Use of Fenfluramine and Phentermine Alone and in Combination." *Archives of Internal Medicine* 144, no. 6 (1984): 1143–1148.

Weintraub, M., P. R. Sundaresan, B. Schuster, G. Ginsberg, M. Madan, A. Balder, E. C. Stein, and L. Byrne. "Long-term Weight Control Study. II (Weeks 34 to 104). An Open-Label Study of Continuous Fenfluramine Plus Phentermine versus Targeted Intermittent Medication as Adjuncts to Behavior Modification, Caloric Restriction, and Exercise." *Clinical Pharmacology & Therapeutics* 51, no. 5 (1992): 595–601.

West, J. A., and A. E. de Looy. "Weight Loss in Overweight Subjects Following Low-Sucrose or Sucrose-Containing Diets." *International Journal of Obesity-Related Metabolic Disorders* 25, no. 8 (2001): 1122–1128.

Wing, R. R. "Behavioral Strategies to Improve Long-term Weight Loss and Maintenance." *Medicine & Health Rhode Island* 82, no. 4 (1999): 123.

Wolfe, B. M., and J. M. Morton. "Weighing In on Bariatric Surgery: Procedure Use, Readmission Rates, and Mortality." *Journal of the American Medical Association* 294, no. 15 (2005): 1960–1963.

Wolfe, S. M., L. D. Sasich, and E. Barbenhenn. "Petition to FDA to Ban the Diet Drug Sibutramine (Meridia)." Washington, DC: U.S. Food and Drug Administration, 2002.

Wylie-Rosett, J. "Fat Substitutes and Health: An Advisory from the Nutrition Committee of the American Heart Association." *Circulation* 105, no. 23 (2002): 2800–2804.

3

Worldwide Perspective

Multinational Scope of Overweight and Obesity

Throughout history, a primary goal of human work was to acquire enough food to prevent starvation. In 2000, a historical moment occurred when the estimate of the number of overweight people in the world exceeded the number of those who were underweight (Gardner and Halweil 2000). The prevalence of obesity and overweight in adults and children is rapidly increasing in most parts of the world. Eating too much food has become a concern, as overweight and obesity have joined underweight, malnutrition, and infectious diseases as serious health issues in developing countries. The World Health Organization (WHO) now describes global obesity, or "globesity," as one of the top 10 risks to human health. There were an estimated 200 million obese people (those with a body mass index, or BMI, of 30 or above) in 1995, but in 2005, more than 400 million people were classified as obese. Experts at WHO predict that, by 2015, the number of obese individuals will exceed 700 million (WHO 2008).

Data on obesity in the developing world are limited, and extreme variability is seen in obesity rates between countries and even within rural and urban areas of the same country. The highest rates seem to occur in the South Pacific. On Nauru, an island approximately 2,500 miles southwest of Hawaii, whose population descended from Polynesian seafarers, 70 percent of the population is classified as obese, up from just 15 percent in the 1960s. In urban Samoa, three-quarters of adults are obese. The body weight increases are not restricted to this region. Overweight and obesity affect 25 to 50 percent of men, women, and children in countries as diverse as Brazil, Germany, and Australia. Even in countries with obesity levels below 5 percent, such as China, Japan, and several African nations, rates are almost 20 percent in some cities. The World Health Organization Global Database on Body Mass, with interactive maps, tables, graphs, and detailed data, is an interesting way to check up-to-date examples of the multinational prevalence of adult underweight, overweight, and obesity in both developed countries and nations in transition.

The Weight Gap: Undernutrition Coexists with Obesity

Historically considered a problem only in the rich countries, overweight and obesity are dramatically increasing in low- and middle-income nations. Experts forecast that the biggest rise in obesity in the coming decades will affect developing countries. It is ironic that beneficial economic developments, such as increased wealth, better health care, and a reduction in subsistence farming, have lead to increased rates of obesity. This increase is taking place in countries that are experiencing a nutrition transition due to changes in diet and lifestyle that result from economic development. It is assumed that a central health problem is undernutrition rather than overnutrition for low- and middle-income countries, and the number of hungry people remains high in spite of global food surplus. Many developing countries now face a "double burden" of disease: Infectious diseases and hunger exist side by side with obesity and overweight within the same country or even within the same household. As an example, the majority of India's citizens are undernourished, yet a growing segment of wealthy Indians is becoming obese (Subramanian and Smith 2006).

The emergence of obesity in developing countries initially primarily affected wealthy people. More recent trends show a shift in prevalence from the higher to the lower socioeconomic level. In 1989, national surveys in Brazil found that obesity in adults was more prevalent in the higher socioeconomic levels.

Ten years later, the lower socioeconomic group had a higher percentage of obese individuals (Caballero 2007). This demographic switch means that the developing world will have to cope with the health problems of populations moving from hunger to obesity in a single generation.

Obesity Becoming More Common among Children

In the United States, the prevalence of childhood overweight tripled between 1980 and 2000 (Ogden et al. 2002). Childhood overweight is not unique to the United States, as it has increased in almost all countries for which data are available. Overall, 1 in 10 children is overweight, and even the youngest are affected. In 2007, an estimated 22 million children *under the age of five years* were overweight throughout the world. More than 75 percent of overweight children live in low- and middle-income countries (WHO 2008). Some remarkable facts about childhood obesity are shared in the following list.

- In Europe childhood obesity is most prevalent in Southern European countries. Using the International Obesity Taskforce's (IOTF) strict assessment methods, researchers found that more than a third of nine-year-olds in mainland Italy and in Sicily were overweight or obese. In Spain, 27 percent of children and adolescents were overweight or obese, while in Crete, nearly 40 percent of children age 12 were overweight (Lobstein et al. 2004).
- Comparison of the rates of childhood overweight from the 1970s to the end of the 1990s showed an increase of 66 percent in the United States and an even larger increase (240 percent) during the same period in Brazil (Lobstein and Baur 2005).
- WHO reported that approximately 25 percent of Australian children and adolescents were overweight or obese— a significant jump from 5 percent in the 1960s (WHO 2008).
- In the United States, national surveys have shown that overweight affects children as young as two to five years old (Ogden et al. 2002).

In 2008, some good news was reported in the United States. After years of steady increases in childhood overweight, data from the Centers for Disease Control and Prevention (CDC) showed that rates of overweight did not increase between 1999–2000 and 2005–2006. Perhaps public health campaigns aimed at raising awareness of childhood overweight may have begun to pay off. Further data collection will tell whether these rates reflect an actual plateau in the number of children becoming overweight or a statistical abnormality. Even if childhood obesity rates are slowing, the number of children who currently have an unhealthy weight remains unacceptably high.

Childhood Weight Categories Not Clear

In general, youth 6 to 17 years of age are classified as children, although the word "children" may also mean individuals 6 to 11 years of age and "adolescents" may define those 12 to 17 years of age. The definition of overweight or obesity for children has been inconsistent. The BMI, used for measuring excess body fat in adults, is a less-effective measure for children. Body fat changes considerably with age and differs between girls and boys. Generally, the BMI of a child is compared with the BMI of a reference population of children of the same sex and age. Children are considered overweight if they weigh more than 95 percent of other children in their height and age group. Based on the CDC pediatric growth charts as described in Chapter 1, overweight is defined as at or above the 95th percentile of BMI for age, and children whose values fall between the 85th and 95th percentile of BMI for age are *at risk for overweight* (Flegal, Wei, and Ogden 2002).

The CDC does not use the term "obese" when referring to body weight in children because of concerns about stigma and embarrassment for children and parents. However, the rest of the world does use that terminology. European researchers classify overweight as at or above the 85th percentile and obesity as a BMI for age exceeding the 95th percentile (Flodmark et al. 2004). These standards, which link children's BMI cutoffs to the accepted adult cutoff points of 25 and 30 kg/m^2 (kilograms per meter squared), were developed in 2000 by the International Association for the Study of Obesity. Countries around the world are now using these standards to estimate the rate of childhood obesity (Cole et al. 2000). In 2007, an expert committee from the

American Medical Association (AMA) recommended a change in U.S. terminology to replace "at risk for overweight" with "overweight" and replace "overweight" with "obese" (Barlow 2007). Another category was proposed to define severe obesity as BMI at or above the 99th percentile.

Studies document an association between elevated childhood BMI and increased risk of chronic disease in adulthood (e.g., Baker, Olsen, and Sorensen 2007). Although optimal levels of BMI for long-term health are not known, the increases in the prevalence of obesity foretells mounting rates of obesity-associated disorders in the future.

Changing Lifestyle and Economic Policies

Obesity has been described as both a medical condition and a lifestyle disorder. No single factor is responsible for its onset, as it is influenced by one's genetic background, personal behavior, and the political and social environment. In both developed and developing nations, the prevalence of numerous obesogenic conditions is increasing. As defined in Chapter 1, "obesogenic" is the term used to describe the worldwide economic and cultural changes that have altered food selection and physical activity in ways that promote weight gain. Though these conditions vary greatly by region, it is possible to identify some common trends. As incomes rise and populations become more urban, traditional diets high in complex carbohydrates are replaced with those containing more fats and sugars. At the same time, less physically demanding work is required due to the increasing use of motorized vehicles, labor-saving technology in the home and at work, and more passive leisure activities.

Globalization of Food Production and Marketing

Economic growth, the globalization of food markets, and urbanization allow greater access to high-fat, high-sugar, energy-dense foods. In the *nutrition transition*, developing nations move away from traditional methods of cultivation and preparation of diets that were based on grains and vegetables to consumption of mass-produced processed foods. A large part of this transition is economic. In general, mass-marketed foods are cheaper, particularly in urban areas, while fresh foods are more expensive. Globalization of agricultural policies has contributed to progressive cost reductions in meat, butter, oils, fats, and sugars, while the relative price of fruit and vegetables has climbed.

As a result of these factors, traditional diets are being replaced with high-calorie meals. In addition, taste plays a role in these dietary shifts. From an evolutionary standpoint, humans prefer foods high in fat and sugar. This preference is the result of an adaptation for endurance in times of famine. Only recently have such foods become so cheap and widely available to most of the world's population that eating them becomes a health liability. Major international and domestic corporations attempt to increase financial growth with marketing designed to convince people to eat more than they actually need. Profitable strategies used in countries around the world include creating foods that are convenient to prepare, making foods available everywhere (including schools and workplaces), encouraging eating out instead of preparing food at home, and providing bigger portions for minimal additional cost. Consumers now make a large part of their diet decisions based on information and encouragement from the food industry.

Move to Cities Reduces Physical Activity

In urban areas, the majority of jobs are comparatively sedentary ones that demand less physical energy than does rural labor. Even on farms, less work is required with increased mechanization. Motorized transport in cities reduces walking or cycling. Urban sprawl, as opposed to traditional compact cities, aggravates the situation in many areas. Urban sprawl with lack of public transportation or pedestrian-friendly options has been positively associated with weight gain. With the associated long distances between home, office, and shops, walking and biking are simply not practical ways of getting around. Without safe bicycle routes and walkways, people find it is necessary to drive to places of work and play. A study in 2004 reported a 6 percent increase in the risk of obesity for every hour spent commuting by car each day (Frank, Andresen, and Schmid 2004). Where public transportation is lacking, people miss out on the exercise they could get from walking to and from bus and train stations.

Gender Effects on Obesity

Gender differences further complicate the factors promoting obesity. As more and more women work away from home, traditional patterns of food preparation are changing in developed and developing countries. With migration to cities, many women begin to work outside the home and have less time to purchase and prepare food. These time challenges make prepared and processed foods, which are often high in fat and sugar and low in fiber, vitamins, and minerals, an easy choice. The tendency to eat outside the home or to buy ready-to-eat or prepared meals is also taking the place of time-consuming cooking with basic ingredients. Children are less likely to see examples of meal preparation in the home, and, as a result, cooking skills and practices may be limited in succeeding generations.

Generally, women tend to have higher rates of obesity than men. In several developing countries, the relationship between socioeconomic status and obesity is positive for men but negative for women. Heavier males and thinner females are often associated with wealth, while the reverse occurs in poor communities. Many minority and lower-income groups associate fatness with prosperity (WHO 2008). Another obesity profile is seen in Eastern Mediterranean countries. In Saudi Arabia, Kuwait, Bahrain, Qatar, and the United Arab Emirates, the obesity percentage among married women ranges from 35 to 75 percent and among married men from 30 to 60 percent. Diets that include fatty foods, inactivity, and multiparity, or the repetition of pregnancy with short intervals between giving birth and pregnancy, boost the obesity rate in this region (Musaiger 2004).

Growing awareness of the negative health effect of the industrial diet is persuading health-conscious people in the United States, Brazil, Thailand, and Chile, for example, to avoid processed foods, improve exercise habits, and go back to a whole-food diet that is low in fat and added sugar and high in whole grains, fruits, and vegetables. A compelling question is whether obesity will become the disease of poverty. People with the most resources will be able to eat nutritious food and maintain proper weight, while the poorest, with less access to healthy food and nutrition education, are increasingly likely to be overweight.

Obesogenic Environment's Influence on Children

Urban children in most countries are exposed to high-calorie foods, increased frequency of eating occasions, and soft drinks replacing water. Fast food is now a staple of many children's diets. Children who consume fast food, as compared with those who do not, have higher caloric intake, including more fat and more sugar (Bowman et al. 2004). The United States has been called a fast food nation. Every day, one out of four Americans eats fast food, and a 2004 study revealed that 30 percent of children eat fast food on a daily basis (Bowman and Vinyard 2004). Most parents provide fast-food meals out of convenience—lack of time leads many people to the drive-through. Money plays a part as well, as fast-food restaurants are often the cheapest option.

Increased calorie consumption is not matched by adequate levels of physical activity in young people. Researchers have found that worldwide urbanization of society is reducing children's physical activity opportunities. For example, fewer children walk or bicycle to school, and school-based physical education has decreased. Thirty years ago, nearly half of American children walked or biked to school; today, less than one in five gets to school under her or his own power (McDonald 2007). The 2005 *Dietary Guidelines for Americans* recommends that children and adolescents engage in at least 60 minutes of physical activity on most days of the week. In analysis conducted on data collected from more than 1,000 children from ethnically and economically diverse backgrounds in the United States, researchers found that, at age nine, more than 90 percent of the children met the recommended level of 60 minutes or more of activity each day. The researchers tracked these children over the years and found that, by age 15, only 31 percent met the recommended level on weekdays, and 17 percent met the recommended level on weekends. On average, boys were more active than girls (Nader et al. 2008).

Children may be spending more time watching television, playing computer games, and performing other sedentary activities at the expense of leisure physical activity and sports (St-Onge, Keller, and Heymsfield 2003). In the United States, young people spend an average of almost 6.5 hours a day with electronic media. That figure represents an increase of more than an hour since 2000. Most of the time is spent with video games and computers. According to a 2005 study by the Kaiser Family Foundation, the typical 8- to 18-year-old lives in a home with an average of 3.6 compact disc or tape players, 3.5 TVs, 3.3 radios, 2.9 video players, 2.1 video game consoles, and 1.5 computers (KFF 2005).

Investigators have hypothesized that electronic media contribute to childhood obesity because sedentary media behavior displaces time that would be spent in physical activity (Epstein and Roemmich 2001). It has also been demonstrated that calorie intake increases with media use. Adolescents engaging in high television and media use eat more fat, sugar, and high-density foods (Robinson 2001). Not all studies have shown a correlation between electronic media use and obesity, however. Past studies have primarily focused on television viewing and did not include computer video games and Internet use. These media encourage young people to be sedentary; however, their impact on eating behavior is presently unknown.

Global Health Risks Associated with Childhood Obesity

In the 1990s, WHO initiated global public awareness campaigns for policy makers, industry, medical professionals, and the general public about the health consequences of obesity. For people everywhere, being overweight and obese carries serious health consequences, from increased risk of premature death to chronic conditions that reduce overall quality of life. Obesity increases the risk of heart disease and stroke, primary causes of death throughout the world (WHO 2008).

Another health impact of global obesity is seen in the fast-rising rates of type 2 diabetes, for which obesity is a key risk factor. According to the International Diabetes Federation, the number of people with diabetes worldwide is more than 150 million, a fivefold increase since 1985 (King, Aubert, and Herman 1998). If current trends continue, significant increases in type 2 diabetes are predicted in China, Latin America, India, and the Middle East in the next decade (WHO 2003).

Researchers are interested in whether children face the same health risks as adults. Studies show a sharp increase in the number of children with type 2 diabetes. The condition was once known as adult-onset diabetes before it started showing up in obese children even before puberty. As with adults, diabetes increases a child's risk for blindness, nerve damage, kidney failure, and cardiovascular disease (Hossain, Kowar, and El Nahas 2007). The IOTF report "Obesity in Children and Young People: A Crisis in Public Health" warned that health consequences of child overweight and obesity may not become evident until adulthood. Studies show that overweight children are more likely to be obese as adults (e.g., Whitaker et al. 1997), and overweight that occurs in childhood is more predictive of later extreme obesity than obesity that begins in adulthood. When increasing numbers of overweight children grow up, experts predict, health care problems will surge. The fact that the American Academy of Pediatrics has recommended cholesterol screening of young children with the possibility of prescribing cholesterol-lowering drugs to prevent cardiovascular disease and the controversial idea that children today may live less healthy and shorter lives than their parents are dramatic examples of the effect obesity has on the health of youth today.

Managing Childhood Overweight and Obesity

Any intervention that reduces positive energy balance (excess calories) will be effective in preventing body fat storage. Obesity management has centered, for the most part, on the two sides of the energy balance equation: energy taken in and energy expended. Dietary strategies for overweight children are similar to those for adults, with treatment goals based on age and risk factors. Most food plans for weight loss emphasize providing age-appropriate food portion sizes, reducing the number of meals eaten outside the home, increasing fruit and vegetable consumption, and structuring meal times and places. Children are similar to adults in that regular exercise provides health benefits even when weight is unchanged. Regular physical activity is critical for the prevention of excess weight gain and weight maintenance.

Weight management involves both short-term medical treatment of established obesity and its complications and long-term prevention strategies. Prevention involves both personal responsibility for weight control and a community-based set of tactics that create environmental support for healthy diets and regular physical activity. Approaches to prevention for individuals include health education, behavior modification, medication, and surgery. Population-based interventions such as requiring menu labeling to show calories, providing attractive fruit and vegetable choices in schools, including those available in the à la carte areas and vending machines, and encouraging physical activity by creating bike and walking paths improve public food and activity environments.

Medical Treatment

Prevention is a primary feature of pediatric medical practice. Along with immunizations and promoting use of automobile safety seats, identification of excessive weight gain can be a routine part of childhood medical examinations. Health care professionals are encouraged to routinely track BMI in children and youth and offer appropriate counseling and guidance to children and their families. Individual behavioral modification and medical treatment are appropriate for children who are already overweight, as early weight management can be a successful tactic for preventing adult obesity. Although pediatricians may be concerned about their patients' obesity, most are not prepared to treat obese children. The AMA has launched a campaign to educate physicians about how to prevent and manage childhood obesity. The goal is to include training as part of undergraduate, graduate, and continuing medical education programs. The AMA Expert Committee recommends that treatment of overweight children be approached in a staged method based upon the child's age, BMI, related comorbidities, progress in treatment, and the child's primary caregiver/family involvement in the process (AMA 2007). The committee created 22 recommendations for health care professionals who provide obesity care to apply in their practices. A complete list of the recommendations can be found in the AMA's "Expert Committee Recommendations on the Assessment, Prevention, and Treatment of Child and Adolescent Overweight and Obesity" (AMA 2007).

Dietary Interventions

One of the recommendations set forth by the AMA is that a dietary assessment should be conducted at each well-child visit. A brief diet history can pinpoint appropriate behaviors to target with explicit goals for diet change. For example, a nutrition risk assessment checklist may identify a patient's high consumption of soda and sweetened beverages. A simple and measurable goal would be to replace soft drinks and juice drinks with water. The frequency of beverage replacement could be negotiated. Similar to treatment of adults, pediatric weight management goals should be realistic and should focus on small, gradual behavioral changes. Rather than restrict food choices, a better plan is to improve food choices.

Clinicians and scientists are learning more about how childhood eating behavior develops and is shaped by the environment; however, no good research exists that suggests how to translate this knowledge into useful practices to prevent obesity. Consensus has been reached that pediatricians should proactively discuss and promote healthy eating behaviors for even the youngest children and encourage parents to provide suitable boundaries and opportunities that encourage healthful eating (AAP 2001).

How to Choose the Best Diet for Children

There is a proper number of calories for each person to eat every day. The number depends on gender, age, and activity level. Children have periods of rapid growth and development, and their energy needs can change rapidly. A child's diet should be like that of the rest of the family, with meals and snacks that offer a variety of nutritious foods (USDA 2005). Government Web sites often offer free information and fact sheets about good nutrition. Country-specific food guides can help show families how to select healthful foods and increase awareness of appropriate portion sizes for any desirable calorie level. Examples of food guides illustrated by graphic displays from various geographic regions are the Food Guide Pyramids of the United States and the

Philippines, the Chinese and Korean Food Guide Pagodas, Canada's rainbow-shaped Guide for Healthy Eating, and the Swedish Food Circle (Painter, Rah, and Lee 2002).

The U.S. Department of Agriculture's "Tips from the Pyramid" fact sheet suggests ways to select nutritious meals and provides clear-cut suggestions for following the Pyramid plans. For instance:

Choose whole-grain foods, such as whole-wheat bread, oatmeal, brown rice, and low-fat popcorn, more often.

Focus on fruits. Eat them at meals and at snack time. Choose fresh, frozen, canned, or dried, but go easy on the fruit juice.

Whole Grains

Bread, cereal, and pasta account for a large part of the carbohydrates most people eat. These starches can be made from whole-grain flours or from refined flours. Whole grains provide fiber, minerals, and vitamins that are lost when a grain is refined. Some examples of whole-grain products and serving sizes are: 1/2 cup of cooked brown rice, whole-wheat pasta, or rolled oats; one slice of 100 percent whole-grain bread; or one 6-inch whole-wheat tortilla.

The advice to limit sweet drinks is important because consumption of juices and sweetened beverages is associated with weight gain. By 14 years of age, 32 percent of girls and 52 percent of boys in the United States are consuming 24 or more ounces of sweetened soft drinks daily. A common 12-ounce serving of a sweetened soft drink contains the equivalent of 10 teaspoons of sugar. Serving sizes of 16, 20, and 32 ounces or more are frequently sold in fast-food outlets or quick shop markets. Not surprisingly, children and adolescents who consume soft drinks regularly have a higher energy intake than those who do not. They are also likely to be overweight or obese (Ludwig, Peterson, and Gortmaker 2001). Even juices made from fresh fruit contain concentrated sugars and calories. Most have little or no fiber, and excessive juice intake can result in unwanted weight gain. The American Academy of Pediatrics has issued these recommendations about juice in children's diets:

- For children ages one to six, intake of fruit juice should be limited to 4 to 6 ounces a day.
- For children 7 to 18, limit juice intake to 8 to 12 ounces a day.

- All children should be encouraged to eat whole fruits. (AAP 2001).

Fruits and Vegetables

The average child in the United States does not consume enough fruits and vegetables. The *Dietary Guidelines for Americans* emphasize that children should eat amounts of fruits and vegetables appropriate for their calorie needs, and choose from a variety each day (USDA 2005). For example, a child who requires 1,500 calories per day should have about 1 cup of vegetables. Fresh, frozen, and canned vegetables all count toward meeting vegetable intake goals. Most fruits and vegetables are low in fat and calories, and they also provide essential vitamins, minerals, fiber, and phytochemicals that promote good health.

Pharmacological Treatment

Data about pharmacological, or drug, therapy for overweight and obesity in children are limited and controversial (Yanovski 2001). In a randomized controlled trial of severe obesity, the drug sibutramine was more effective than behavior therapy alone; however, the medication is associated with side effects including increased heart rate and blood pressure (Berkowitz et al. 2003). The fat-blocking drug orlistat is approved for use in adolescents, and a study of 12- to 16-year-old obese boys and girls showed that orlistat, in combination with diet, exercise, and behavior modification, significantly enhanced weight loss compared with placebo. The use of orlistat for one year did not show major safety issues, although gastrointestinal side effects were more common in the orlistat group (Chanoine et al. 2005).

Surgical Treatment

Rising numbers of youth with a BMI of 50 or above, or a BMI of 40 or above with severe comorbidities such as type 2 diabetes, are undergoing bariatric surgery. The AMA advises that surgical therapy be reserved for full-grown adolescents with treatment by experienced multidisciplinary teams who can provide comprehensive medical and psychological care. Reviews of trials of weight-loss surgery indicate that it is an effective and safe alternative for obese adolescents who have not responded to medical therapy. Long-term data, including information on malabsorption of critical nutrients and effects on maturation, are unknown. More study is needed to definitively accept this therapy for obesity in adolescents (Xanthakos, Daniels, and Inge 2006).

Health Care Delivery Systems

Contemporary health care often focuses on short-term interventions and does not have policies or employ strategies to meet the long-term needs of overweight children and their families. Effective childhood weight management relies upon a comprehensive approach that targets the individual, the family, and the environmental influences. These time-consuming models also require changes in how obesity treatment and prevention services are financed. Long-term weight-management programs are beyond the reach of people who lack personal financial resources or whose insurance does not cover obesity treatment. In many countries, including the United States, changes in health care systems are needed to meet needs of long-term weight management for both adults and children.

Prevention

Childhood is a period during which lifelong habits are formed and overweight and obesity, as well as their related diseases, are theoretically preventable. It makes sense to initiate obesity prevention programs for children, rather than focus on treating the disease only after it already exists. Unlike most adults, children and adolescents cannot choose the environment in which they live or the food they eat. They also have a limited ability to understand the long-term consequences of their behavior. For these reasons, they require adult consideration and help to prevent overweight and obesity. In town meetings sponsored by Shaping America's Youth, a nationwide initiative to identify and centralize obesity prevention programs for children and adolescents, Executive Director Dr. David McCarron has asserted that obesity cannot be blamed solely on fast-food restaurants, computer makers, or parents. He describes obesity as a multifaceted problem that requires communities to take responsibility and join together to resolve it.

Coordinated Strategies for Childhood Obesity Prevention

In the United States, numerous state and local prevention programs are in place to increase physical activity and promote healthful eating among children and youth. Current interventions generally are not part of a national, focused effort to combat obesity. In 2005, an Institute of Medicine (IOM) report, *Preventing Childhood Obesity: Health in the Balance*, offered a guide for coordinating contributions from government, schools, industry, media, and families. Three years later, in collaboration with the Robert Wood Johnson Foundation, the IOM established the Standing Committee on Childhood Obesity Prevention. This committee will remain in place to consistently assess America's progress toward meeting the recommendations from the earlier plan and to make suggestions for integrating ideas and programs from government, academia, and corporate sectors. Progress toward organizing the federal and state governments' existing childhood obesity prevention programs was made in 2007 when the U.S. Department of Health and Human Services created the Childhood Overweight and Obesity Prevention Initiative. In remarks by First Lady Laura Bush promoting the initiative, she agreed that parents, government officials, and community and education leaders must work together to improve children's health. And she promised that "Our government is working to address one of the greatest dangers to America's young people: childhood overweight and obesity" (Bush 2007).

Global Collaboration to Combat Childhood Obesity

Obesity may be overlooked as a serious health problem in developing countries where policy makers are still focusing on issues of undernutrition, but many nations are increasing obesity prevention programs for children. To be successful, these plans, which encourage children to eat a healthful diet and engage in physical activity, require commitment from political leaders. The prime ministers, kings, presidents, and high-ranking officials within ministries of health can facilitate the political agenda and resource allocation. Their commitment should include a formal, public statement that cites obesity prevention as a priority and provides national goals and strategic action plans created for each country. For example, leaders in China, which will soon have the highest number of people in the world with cardiovascular disease, would need to formulate prevention programs for the nation's particular conditions. Professor Chen Chunming from the Chinese Center for Disease Control and Prevention says, "We need a country-specific strategy for China based on the current situation of the food industry and the food market and of people's dietary patterns, which are different from elsewhere" (Burslem 2004).

To promote healthy lifestyles for adults and children in all countries, WHO developed the Global Strategy on Diet, Physical Activity and Health (DPAS), which was endorsed by the 57th World Health Assembly in May 2004. DPAS aims to reduce noncommunicable diseases such as obesity, diabetes, and cardiovascular disease by modifying risk factors such as unhealthy diet and physical inactivity. The advice from DPAS is not complicated. The basic guidelines suggest increasing consumption of fruit and vegetables, legumes, whole grains, and nuts; limiting energy intake from fats; limiting intake of sugars; and being physically active. The physical activity guideline is perhaps the most challenging for city dwellers because its goal of at least 60 minutes of regular, moderate- to vigorous-intensity exercise each day that is age appropriate and involves a variety of activities is often difficult for them to achieve.

As obesity prevention plans will require fundamental social and political changes, DPAS also provides detailed lists of responsibilities of key stakeholders including WHO, international partners, nongovernmental organizations, and the private sector. DPAS offers resources to assist different stakeholders in its implementation. Frameworks such as those shown below can be found in the "Implementation Toolbox" section on the WHO DPAS Web site, http://www.who.int/dietphysicalactivity/en/.

- **A Framework to Monitor and Evaluate Implementation** provides methods to measure progress when DPAS recommendations are implemented.
- **The WHO/Food and Agriculture Organization Fruit and Vegetables for Health framework** guides the development of cost-efficient and effective interventions for

promotion of fruit and vegetable production and
consumption.

- **The Move for Health Initiative** facilitates development of
long-term national and local physical activity policies and
programs to increase physical activity in all domains (leisure time, transport, work) and settings (school, community, home, workplace).

Possibly stimulated by the thinking that created DPAS, an
increasing number of nations have created health policies related
to healthful nutrition and activity. The Netherlands adopted a
national health care prevention policy in 2004, identifying
obesity as one of the three priorities, along with smoking and
diabetes. In early 2005, Spain adopted a national strategy for
nutrition, physical activity, and prevention of obesity. The same
year, the Slovenian Parliament approved its National Nutrition
Policy. This policy was one of the first examples of high-level
political support for a national nutrition policy in Central and
Eastern Europe (WHO 2006). Several countries, including Brazil,
India, and China, have initiated monitoring programs related to
obesity and nutrition.

The value of these programs cannot be determined yet, as
they are still in their early stages and few data are available. Pre-
liminary experience suggests that a population-based approach
to modifying the obesogenic environment is worth a try because
the customary practice of expecting individuals to take total
responsibility for their diet and exercise choices has failed so
far. WHO recognizes that global childhood obesity is linked not
only to children's behavior but also to social and economic development and policies regulating agriculture, urban planning,
food processing, marketing, and education. Ensuring successful
obesity prevention strategies will take a coordinated effort
among such diverse groups as politicians and legislators, city
planners, schools, food producers, advertisers, parents, and the
medical community.

Goals for Government, Schools, Media and Marketing, Parents, and Researchers

Government

Almost every aspect of government can have an influence on its
citizens' nutrition and activity practices. The IOM suggests that

the federal government be responsible for coordinating federal obesity prevention actions and programs, setting standards for foods and beverages sold in schools, establishing principles regarding advertising and marketing to children and youth, and providing funding for obesity prevention research (IOM 2005). Activists in many countries campaign for the development of schools that promote physical activity, for food and agricultural policies that stimulate availability and affordability of fruits and vegetables, and for urban planning that has built-in ways to encourage physical activity.

A key role of government is to regulate the urban environment to create towns and cities that can sustain and support good health. Access to safe spaces for play is particularly important for children. This need must translate into urban planning that includes building parks and playgrounds and bike paths and pedestrian malls, restrains suburban sprawl, funds public transportation, and makes automobile use less attractive and less necessary. Urban environment and community design can have a great impact on nutrition. The lack of full-service grocery stores, farmers' markets, or community gardens in many urban centers sharply reduces access to affordable fresh fruits and vegetables. Opportunities to eat fast, energy-dense foods increase when the presence of fast-food outlets is pervasive and unregulated. Further, the location of schools can enhance or undermine children's physical activity. One study found that the primary reason that children do not walk or bike to school is because their school is too far away. Other concerns included too much traffic, no safe route, and crime in the neighborhood (CDC 2002).

Schools

Schools offer many opportunities for obesity prevention. They are the place where children spend a large part of their lives. Most schools serve at least one meal a day, and consequently they are able to set positive examples that help children establish healthful eating habits. In addition, schools can encourage children to get exercise and can address nutrition and healthy lifestyles in the school curriculum. The IOM suggested that schools can have an impact on students' well-being by:

- Improving the nutritional quality of foods and beverages served and sold in schools and as part of school-related activities

- Increasing opportunities for frequent, more intensive, and engaging physical activity during and after school
- Developing, implementing, and evaluating innovative programs for teaching about wellness, healthful eating, and physical activity. (IOM 2005)

The ways in which diets and activity can be improved are exemplified by a number of communities. In Berkeley, California, a portion of the produce for cafeteria meals comes from student-managed gardens (Ozer 2007). In Singapore, the Trim and Fit Scheme reduced obesity among children by up to 50 percent through changes in school catering and better nutrition and physical education for students and teachers. Overweight children were expected to do rigorous exercise during breaks and before and after school until they lost a required amount of weight. Although the program did result in weight loss, parents complained that their children were being singled out and teased by classmates. In March 2007, Trim and Fit was ended and the program was to be replaced with a plan that encourages a healthful lifestyle for all schoolchildren instead of just the overweight ones. Singaporean health officials and educators believe that the school-based intervention can benefit a generation growing up on fast food and computer games (AP 2007).

In the United States, school meals are available both from the U.S. Department of Agriculture school breakfast and lunch programs and from commercial venders that provide food for cafeterias, vending machines, and snack bars. Government-provided meals must meet federal nutrition standards, but commercial foods are exempt from those requirements. Some school administrators contend that budget pressures force them to sell popular, but nutritionally lacking, foods. In response to schools being criticized for offering children fast food and soda while scaling back physical education classes and recess, some states are limiting sales of soft drinks and commercial foods of low nutritional value. Schools need adequate resources from federal and state government funding to create school environments that provide adequate physical activity and healthful foods and beverages for students.

On the global level, DPAS states, "School policies and programs should support the adoption of healthy diets and physical activity" (WHO 2003). As part of the implementation of DPAS, in 2008 WHO developed the School Policy Framework to guide policy makers at national and local levels in the development and implementation of policies that promote healthy eating and physical activity in schools.

Marketing

Among the various environment influences on children and youth, the media in its multiple forms have assumed a central role. Advertising and marketing messages reach young consumers through radio, television, magazines, computers, and cell phones. Although children's food choices are strongly influenced by their families, they are increasingly making decisions based on advertising. Children are not "rational consumers"— that is, they do not evaluate information critically and weigh the future consequences of their actions. When vigorous marketing of unhealthful foods is aimed directly at children, blaming children for eating those foods is illogical. They need education from parents, schools, government, and advertisers to help them make healthful choices. If America's young people are to avoid a future of diet-related chronic diseases, they should limit those high-calorie snacks, fast foods, and sugar-sweetened drinks the focus of which comprise the majority of advertisements targeted to children and youth.

Researchers report that children view an average of 40,000 television ads a year. A child watching Saturday morning television may see one food commercial every five minutes, with most featuring such energy-dense, minimally nutritious foods as candy, sugared cereal, and fast food (Kotz and Story 1994). Advertising does influence what foods children want and therefore what parents buy; companies would not spend millions of dollars in advertising if it did not work. In 1997, the food industry was the second largest advertiser in the United States, with television as the most popular medium. Importantly, these advertisement dollars are spent disproportionately on highly processed and packaged foods. During that year, nearly seven times as much money was spent advertising confectionery and snacks (e.g., candy, gum, mints, cookies, crackers, nuts, chips) than was spent advertising fruits, vegetables, grains, and beans. In the same year, the food industry spent $7 billion on advertising, more than 20 times the $333 million spent by the U.S. Department of Agriculture on nutrition education that year (Gallo 1998).

International studies have suggested that overweight among children is related to the quantity of advertising on children's television. A significant association was found between childhood overweight and the number of advertisements per hour on children's television in the United States, Australia, and eight European countries. The authors proposed that these findings support recommendations to reduce children's exposure to marketing practices that typically encourage high-calorie, low-nutrient foods (Lobstein and Baur 2005).

How marketing influences children and youth is the focus of the IOM report *Food Marketing to Children and Youth: Threat or Opportunity?* The report provides a comprehensive review of the scientific evidence on the influence of food marketing on diets and diet-related health of children and youth. The study was requested by the U.S. Congress and sponsored by the CDC. The report states that "Industry should develop and strictly adhere to marketing and advertising guidelines that minimize the risk of obesity in children and youth" (IOM 2006). Responsible marketing messages that encourage a healthy diet would depict food in reasonable portion sizes, not portray overeating as exciting or desirable. They would promote products that are consistent with the *Dietary Guidelines for Americans*, including fruits, vegetables, whole grains, and low-fat milk. They would not portray healthful foods negatively. Marketers are also encouraged to expand nutrition information at the point of purchase and on food labels.

The concerns related to marketing influence are not unique to the United States. Several countries have instituted restrictions on food and beverage advertising to children. Marketing campaigns and price incentives have an important impact on food purchasing patterns in developing countries, where as much as 60 percent of household income is spent on food. A WHO forum on marketing food and nonalcoholic beverages to children met in Oslo, Norway, in 2006. The members reviewed the current influences of marketing on children's food preferences. They discussed how to get all stakeholders involved in managing and limiting negative influences of marketing and advertising on children's dietary choices. Meeting participants recommended that WHO should:

(i) support national action to protect children from marketing by substantially reducing the volume and impact of commercial promotion of energy-dense, micronutrient-poor foods and beverages to children; (ii) address issues such as cross-border television advertising and global promotional activities; and, (iii) consider the development of an international code on the marketing of food and beverages to children. (WHO 2006)

These conclusions and recommendations reflected the opinions of the meeting participants and were not endorsed by WHO. WHO is developing its own, similar recommendations for national action and principles of good practices on the marketing of food and nonalcoholic beverages to children. Publication is expected in 2010.

In 2008, world obesity experts called on food and soft drink manufacturers to adopt international standards to control the marketing of "junk food" to children. Professor Arne Astrup, president of the International Association for the Study of Obesity, an association that represents 10,000 obesity specialists in 55 countries, proposed tough measures to cut the promotion of sweetened soft drinks and food products that are high in fats, sugar, and salt (Rigby 2008). The proposed code would ban all advertising of junk food and sweetened soft drinks to children under 16 on television before 9:00 p.m. Using celebrities and cartoons for this kind of advertising, already forbidden in Ireland, would also be prohibited.

Health advocates who believe the food industry advertising, marketing, and pricing practices contribute to childhood overweight and obesity urge such measures as requiring nutrition information on restaurant and fast-food menus. They also support restrictions on ads aimed at children. Often these initiatives encounter strong opposition from food manufacturers and consumer groups that are concerned about the effects of these limitations on their civil liberties. The challenge will be to find ways that all parties that have an interest in the issue will embrace obesity prevention and to make the food and beverage industry part of the solution.

Parents

An interaction between similar genetic background and environment makes obesity seem inescapable for some, as it "runs in the family." Obese children under three years of age without obese parents are at low risk for obesity in adulthood, but among children under 10 years of age, parental obesity more than doubles the risk of adult obesity (Whitaker et al. 1997). Although the greatest influence parents have on child overweight and obesity is genetic, genetics alone cannot explain the recent increases in obesity throughout the world. Parents may transmit susceptibility, but an obesogenic environment must be present for obesity to occur. Determining how much "nature" or "nurture" is responsible for child overweight can be difficult. Genetics and conscious behavior interact when both parents and children gain weight in households where energy-dense foods are freely available. Similarly, children's physical activity is influenced by how active their parents are.

Often, the best defense against child obesity is strong parental intervention and lifestyle change made by the whole family. In most cases, the child is mimicking the parent's approach to physical activities and healthy eating patterns. Preventive interventions should occur at an age when children's eating habits are more easily influenced by parents and by environmental changes. Young children have little control over their environment, which includes the availability of food and family activities. Because parents do have great influence over these factors, preventive interventions may be most effective if targeted toward parents of those children.

To help children maintain a healthy weight and lifestyle, parents and caregivers can aim for these goals:

- Be positive role models for their children regarding eating habits
- Promote healthful eating behaviors for the entire family
- Provide an environment that makes healthful food and beverage choices easy for children
- Educate children to make healthful decisions about frequency, portion size, and types of foods and beverages to consume
- Encourage everyday physical activity

Serve as Role Models
Helping children adopt healthy eating habits and be physically more active is a family affair. When children see adults eating a variety of nutritious foods, they will be more likely to want to eat them, too. Studies demonstrate that child dietary behavior is strongly influenced by parent role modeling, and, whether apparent or not, research does show that parents continue to be role

models for adolescents (Brown and Ogden 2004). Perhaps the single most effective way to change a child's diet is for adults to set a good example. Parents can be challenged to teach children what to eat, how much to eat, and when to eat and to be consistent and set limits when necessary.

Parents provide a positive role model by:

- Eating healthy, nutritious foods
- Controlling portion sizes
- Limiting treats and high-calorie snacks

Parents can prevent children from picking up unhealthy habits by avoiding:

- Skipping breakfast
- Eating a late dinner or snacking before going to sleep
- Eating in front of the television
- Eating when they are not hungry because of boredom or stress

Involve the Entire Family

Children are not able to change their eating habits by themselves. They need the help and support of their families and other caregivers. Thus, successful prevention and treatment of childhood obesity starts at home (Plourde 2006). The entire family should be involved in health behavior change, including siblings, grandparents, and other caregivers. Successful childhood obesity prevention and treatment depends on parents and other family members to create a home environment that makes healthful eating a priority. Each family member can contribute. Even young children can help with washing fruits and vegetables, setting the table, or stirring ingredients.

Create an Environment That Makes Healthful Eating Easy

Children usually do not do the grocery shopping or food preparation themselves. Parents are the food policy makers at home. A parent's responsibility is to buy healthy groceries, serve nutritious food, and to establish a routine for eating. Parents create a healthy environment when they:

- Avoid arguments about high-fat, high-sugar foods by not bringing them into the house

- Offer whole-grain foods with meals and snacks
- Serve water when a child is thirsty
- Reduce the number of meals eaten out at fast-food and other restaurants
- Sit down together for family meals

Establishing a routine for eating means there is a set time for breakfast, lunch, dinner, and snacks. Most children like to have a schedule, and they become hungry at regular times. Consistent meal times are vital to fostering a healthy response to hunger and satiety signals. With irregular meal times or constant eating or drinking, children may lose the ability to recognize internal signals of hunger and fullness. Studies show that the more families eat together, the more likely older children and adolescents will consume fruits, vegetables, grains, and calcium-rich foods (e.g., Gillman et al. 2000).

Educate Children to Select Nutritious Foods at Home and Away from Home

Children are more apt to choose healthy meals when they are involved in meal planning, shopping, and food preparation. Parental guidance in food choices is necessary, but equally important is teaching children consumer skills to help them make informed choices. As they mature, children begin to make their own choices at school and in other away-from-home settings. Children of all ages, but particularly adolescents, imitate their peers. Adolescent food habits can be negatively affected when they consume "popular" foods such as potato chips, sodas, and candy. These foods provide lots of carbohydrates and fat and little protein, vitamins, or minerals—except for salt. When parents withhold favorite foods, children crave those foods and tend to overeat when they do have access to them (Faith et al. 2004). Teens may turn to dieting methods to lose or control weight, cutting out whole groups of foods (like grain products), skipping meals, and fasting. These methods leave out important foods necessary for growth and health. Other weight-loss practices such as smoking, self-induced vomiting, or using diet pills or laxatives are linked with serious long-term health problems. Unhealthy dieting can actually cause weight gain if it leads to a cycle of eating very little and then overeating or binging on food. Unhealthy dieting also can put adolescents at greater risk for emotional problems. Parents and responsible adults can emphasize that the best way to lose weight is to eat the right amounts of healthful foods and be physically active.

Encourage Everyday Physical Activity

Like adults, kids need daily physical activity. The *Dietary Guidelines for Americans* recommends at least an hour of exercise daily for children and teenagers and 30 minutes a day for adults. The activity does not have to happen all at once; several 10- or even 5-minute periods of activity throughout the day accomplish this goal. Children who are not used to being active can be encouraged to start with any amount they can do and build up to 60 minutes a day. A pre-adolescent child's body is not ready for adult-style physical activity, so children should not be encouraged to participate in activities such as long jogs or lifting heavy weights. Physical activities that kids choose to do on their own often result in the best outcomes (WIN 2008).

Tips for parents from the National Institutes of Health (NIH) Weight Information Network include:

Set a good example. If your child sees that you are physically active and that you have fun doing it, he or she is more likely to be active throughout life.

Encourage your child to join a sports team or class, such as soccer, dance, basketball, or gymnastics at school or at your local community or recreation center.

Be sensitive to your child's needs. If your child feels uncomfortable participating in activities like sports, help her or him find physical activities that are fun and not embarrassing, such as playing tag with friends or siblings, jumping rope, or dancing to his or her favorite music.

Be active together as a family. Assign active chores such as making the beds, washing the car, or vacuuming. Plan active outings such as a trip to the zoo, a family bike ride, or a walk through a local park.

Limit screen time. The more hours a day children and teens spend in front of a TV, video, or computer screen, the more likely they are to be overweight (WIN 2008).

We Can! (Ways to Enhance Children's Activity and Nutrition) is a science-based program and Web site developed by NIH that offers the following tips for parents:

- Limit screen time to no more than two hours a day.
- Do not put a TV in your child's bedroom.

- Make screen time, active time by doing simple exercises during commercial breaks.
- Take a family walk or play ball at the park instead of turning on the TV (WeCan! 2008).

Parents and others can download a free screen time log to help assess the amount of time children spend watching TV, playing video games, or using the computer for recreational purposes (WeCan! 2008).

Parents of obese children face complex challenges, and it may be difficult for working parents to find the time or energy to cook nutritious meals or supervise outdoor playtime. Regardless of ability to achieve the diet and exercise interventions, parents can send the overall message that they not only love and accept their children as they are but also want to support them in being healthy through making healthful food choices and being physically active.

Research

Despite worldwide concern about obesity prevention, no one is sure which policies and programs will actually reduce adult and childhood weight gain. Given the lack of carefully controlled studies, researchers cannot yet establish conclusively that more access to recreation, more active commuting, or cutting out fast food will reduce rates of obesity. More research is needed on a national and an international scale. The misconception that obesity is a problem afflicting only affluent nations and households may be holding back needed research in poorer countries. New international prevention strategies should be tested with consideration of how the nutrition transition affects diets and physical activity among individuals in developing countries.

The lack of definitive research has meant that health care providers and policy makers do not have the kind of detailed information they need to evaluate what might work to reverse obesity trends. An important goal for researchers is to discover effective interventions, particularly for children, which may decrease the risk that they will become obese later in life. The prevalence of overweight in the preschool child population has seen a large increase in the last 20 years (Summerbell et al. 2005), creating an urgent need to reevaluate previous interventions and establish new practice guidelines for practitioners. In 2006, the Robert Wood Johnson Foundation requested that IOM have an expert committee examine progress in preventing childhood obesity in the United States. The resulting report, *Progress in Preventing Childhood Obesity: How Do We Measure Up?* presented specific actions for childhood obesity prevention. One particularly telling point it makes is that lack of a system for monitoring and evaluating progress has reduced the ability to identify, apply, and circulate the lessons learned (IOM 2008). The committee strongly encouraged ongoing surveillance and monitoring systems to track effectiveness of existing policies and nutrition programs, such as feeding programs, and assessing their impact on child health. Because the obesity epidemic is a serious public health problem, it compels immediate action to reduce its prevalence as well as its health and social consequences. The IOM committee felt strongly that actions should be taken now based on the best *available* evidence—as opposed to waiting for the best *possible* evidence.

NIH is a key contributor and the primary funding body for research into the causes, consequences, and prevention of childhood obesity. Currently, NIH funds more than 90 percent of all obesity research in the United States. The *Strategic Plan for NIH Obesity Research* was published in 2004 to provide a guide for coordinating obesity research activities across NIH. The plan's goals, and strategies for achieving them, include:

- Research toward preventing and treating obesity through lifestyle modification
- Research toward preventing and treating obesity through pharmacologic, surgical, or other medical approaches
- Research toward breaking the link between obesity and its associated health conditions
- Cross-cutting research topics, including health disparities, technology, fostering of interdisciplinary research teams, investigator training, translational research, and education/outreach efforts (NIH 2004).

Because environmental, social, economic, and behavioral factors act with genetic susceptibility to contribute to obesity, NIH supports a broad range of investigation. The scope of obesity research includes molecular, genetic, behavioral, environmental, clinical, and epidemiologic studies. The National Cancer Institute, National Human Genome Research Institute, National Institute on Aging, Office of Behavioral and Social

Sciences Research, Office of Dietary Supplements, and Office of Research on Women's Health are some of the institutes that carry out obesity research.

As diverse as these institutes are, most of the funded grants for childhood obesity research focus on diet and physical activity, and very few examine pharmacological or surgical interventions. In 2007, NIH initiated research that would evaluate the benefits and risks of bariatric surgery in adolescents. The Teen Longitudinal Assessment of Bariatric Surgery (Teen-LABS) study was designed to determine if surgery is an appropriate treatment option for extremely overweight teens. During the five-year study, researchers will compare data from 200 adolescents scheduled for bariatric surgery with data from 200 adults who had bariatric surgery. "We know that bariatric surgery is not an easy way out for teens to control weight. They will still need to eat less food and exercise more," says Mary Horlick, MD, project scientist for Teen-LABS at NIH. "We hope to learn whether or not bariatric surgery is suitable for teens and if it will help them remain at a healthy weight over the long-term" (NIH 2007). To participate in the study, young males and females must be 12 to 18 years old and have been approved for bariatric surgery. To justify this invasive surgical procedure, which carries lifelong consequences, most pediatric weight-management experts agree that candidates for surgery should have a BMI of at least 40 as well as an identifiable physical or psychosocial comorbidity of obesity. This standard is in contrast to NIH guidelines for adults, which specify that a BMI of at least 40 without comorbidities justifies this surgery. As with adults, teens should have already tried other noninvasive approaches, and surgery should not be the first intervention.

There is currently no conclusive evidence that changes in the nutrition environment will reduce rates of obesity. Nations, states, and individuals are trying new obesity prevention strategies. These practices can teach about effective ways to reduce child obesity, but to realize their full promise, the policies, programs, and plans must be carefully evaluated. A prerequisite for any effective public health intervention is a solid base of knowledge about what does actually improve health. Building this knowledge base will take time, attention, and funding; however, it is essential to halting the rise in adult and childhood obesity.

Conclusion

Throughout the world, prevention of adult and childhood overweight and obesity presents community-wide as well as individual challenges. To tackle the obesity epidemic, all communities should be healthful places to live, and healthy choices should be easy to make for everyone. Obesity prevention demands a cultural shift, one in which healthy environments, physical activity, and healthy eating become the norm.

References

American Academy of Pediatrics (AAP). "The Use and Misuse of Fruit Juice in Pediatrics." *Pediatrics* 107, no. 5 (2001): 1210–1213.

American Medical Association (AMA). "Appendix: Expert Committee Recommendations on the Assessment, Prevention, and Treatment of Child and Adolescent Overweight and Obesity." 2007. [Online information; retrieved 1/8/09.] http://www.ama-assn.org/ama1/pub/upload/mm/433/ped_obesity_recs.pdf.

Associated Press (AP). "Singapore to Scrap Anti-Obesity Program." *Washington Post*, March 20, 2007.

Baker, J. L., L. W. Olsen, and T. I. Sorensen. "Childhood Body-Mass Index and the Risk of Coronary Heart Disease in Adulthood." *New England Journal of Medicine* 357, no. 23 (2007): 2329–2337.

Barlow, S. E. "Expert Committee Recommendations Regarding the Prevention, Assessment, and Treatment of Child and Adolescent Overweight and Obesity: Summary Report." *Pediatrics* 120, Suppl. 4 (2007): S164–S192.

Berkowitz, R. I., T. A. Wadden, A. M. Tershakovec, and J. L. Cronquist. "Behavior Therapy and Sibutramine for the Treatment of Adolescent Obesity: A Randomized Controlled Trial." *Journal of the American Medical Association* 289, no. 14 (2003): 1805–1812.

Bowman, S. A., S. L. Gortmaker, C. B. Ebbeling, M. A. Pereira, and D. S. Ludwig. "Effects of Fast-Food Consumption on Energy Intake and Diet Quality among Children in a National Household Survey." *Pediatrics* 113, no. 1, Pt. 1 (2004): 112–118.

Bowman, S. A., and B. T. Vinyard. "Fast Food Consumption of U.S. Adults: Impact on Energy and Nutrient Intakes and Overweight Status." *Journal of the American College of Nutrition* 23, no. 2 (2004): 163–168.

Brown, R., and J. Ogden. "Children's Eating Attitudes and Behaviour: A Study of the Modelling and Control Theories of Parental Influence." *Health Education Research* 19, no. 3 (2004): 261–271.

Burslem, Chris. "The Changing Face of Malnutrition." *IFPRI Forum* October (2004).

Bush, L. "Mrs. Bush's Remarks at the 2007 National Prevention and Health Promotion Summit." 2007. [Online news release; retrieved 1/8/09.] http://www.whitehouse.gov/news/releases/2007/11/20071127-3.html.

Caballero, B. "The Global Epidemic of Obesity: An Overview." *Epidemiologic Reviews* 29 (2007): 1–5.

Centers for Disease Control and Prevention (CDC). "Barriers to Children Walking and Biking to School—United States, 1999." *Morbidity and Mortality Weekly Report* 51, no. 32 (2002):701–704.

Cole, T. J., M. C. Bellizzi, K. M. Flegal, and W. H. Dietz. "Establishing a Standard Definition for Child Overweight and Obesity Worldwide: International Survey." *British Medical Journal* 320, no. 7244 (2000): 1240–1243.

Epstein, L. H., and J. N. Roemmich. "Reducing Sedentary Behavior: Role in Modifying Physical Activity." *Exercise and Sport Sciences Reviews* 29, no. 3 (2001): 103–108.

Faith, M. S., R. I. Berkowitz, V. A. Stallings, J. Kerns, M. Storey, and A. J. Stunkard. "Parental Feeding Attitudes and Styles and Child Body Mass Index: Prospective Analysis of a Gene-Environment Interaction." *Pediatrics* 114, no. 4 (2004): e429–e436.

Flegal, K. M., R. Wei, and C. Ogden. "Weight-for-Stature Compared with Body Mass Index-for-Age Growth Charts for the United States from the Centers for Disease Control and Prevention." *American Journal of Clinical Nutrition* 75, no. 4 (2002): 761–766.

Flodmark, C. E., I. Lissau, L. A. Moreno, A. Pietrobelli, and K. Widhalm. "New Insights into the Field of Children and Adolescents' Obesity: The European Perspective." *International Journal of Obesity-Related Metabolic Disorders* 28, no. 10 (2004): 1189–1196.

Frank, L. D., M. A. Andresen, and T. L. Schmid. "Obesity Relationships with Community Design, Physical Activity, and Time Spent in Cars." *American Journal of Preventive Medicine* 27, no. 2 (2004): 87–96.

Gallo, A. E. "Food Advertising in the United States. America's Eating Habits: Changes and Consequences." Washington, DC: Food and Rural Economics Division, Economic Research Service, U.S. Department of Agriculture, 1998.

Gardner, G., and B. Halweil. "Overfed and Underfed: The Global Epidemic of Malnutrition." Worldwatch Paper 150. Washington, DC: Worldwatch Institute, 2000.

Gillman, M. W., S. L. Rifas-Shiman, A. L. Frazier, H. R. Rockett, C. A. Camargo, Jr., A. E. Field, C. S. Berkey, and G. A. Colditz. "Family Dinner and Diet Quality among Older Children and Adolescents." *Archives of Family Medicine* 9, no. 3 (2000): 235–240.

Hossain, P., B. Kawar, and M. El Nahas. "Obesity and Diabetes in the Developing World—a Growing Challenge." *New England Journal of Medicine* 356, no. 3 (2007): 213–215.

Institute of Medicine (IOM). *Preventing Childhood Obesity: Health in the Balance*, xix. Washington, DC: National Academies Press, 2005.

Institute of Medicine (IOM). *Food Marketing to Children and Youth: Threat or Opportunity?* Washington, DC: National Academies Press, 2006.

Institute of Medicine (IOM). *Progress in Preventing Childhood Obesity: How Do We Measure Up?* Washington, DC: National Academies Press, 2008.

Kaiser Family Foundation (KFF). "Generation M: Media in the Lives of 8 to 18 Year-Olds." 2005. [Online information; retrieved 1/8/09.] www.kff.org/entmedia/entmedia030905pkg.cfm.

King, H., R. E. Aubert, and W. H. Herman. "Global Burden of Diabetes, 1995–2025: Prevalence, Numerical Estimates, and Projections." *Diabetes Care* 21, no. 9 (1998): 1414–1431.

Kotz, K., and M. Story. "Food Advertisements During Children's Saturday Morning Television Programming: Are They Consistent with Dietary Recommendations?" *Journal of the American Dietetic Association* 94, no. 11 (1994): 1296–1300.

Lobstein, T., and L. A. Baur. "Policies to Prevent Childhood Obesity in the European Union." *European Journal of Public Health* 15, no. 6 (2005): 576–579.

Lobstein, T., L. Baur, R. Uauy, and IASO International Obesity Taskforce. "Obesity in Children and Young People: A Crisis in Public Health." *Obesity Reviews* 5, Suppl. 1 (2004): 4–104.

Ludwig, D. S., K. E. Peterson, and S. L. Gortmaker. "Relation between Consumption of Sugar-sweetened Drinks and Childhood Obesity: A Prospective, Observational Analysis." *Lancet* 357, no. 9255 (2001): 505–508.

McDonald, N. C. "Active Transportation to School: Trends among U.S. Schoolchildren, 1969–2001." *American Journal of Preventive Medicine* 32, no. 6 (2007): 509–516.

Musaiger, A. O. "Overweight and Obesity in the Eastern Mediterranean Region: Can We Control It?" *Eastern Mediterranean Health Journal* 10, no. 6 (2004): 789–793.

Nader, P. R., R. H. Bradley, R. M. Houts, S. L. McRitchie, and M. O'Brien. "Moderate-to-Vigorous Physical Activity from Ages 9 to 15 Years." *Journal of the American Medical Association* 300, no. 3 (2008): 295–305.

National Institutes of Health (NIH). *Strategic Plan for NIH Obesity Research*. Bethesda, MD: National Institutes of Health, 2004.

National Institutes of Health (NIH). "NIH Launches Study to Assess Bariatric Surgery in Adolescents." 2007. [Online news release; retrieved 1/8/09.] http://www.nih.gov/news/pr/apr2007/niddk-16.htm.

Ogden, C. L., R. J. Kuczmarski, K. M. Flegal, Z. Mei, S. Guo, R. Wei, L. M. Grummer-Strawn, L. R. Curtin, A. F. Roche, and C. L. Johnson. "Centers for Disease Control and Prevention 2000 Growth Charts for the United States: Improvements to the 1977 National Center for Health Statistics Version." *Pediatrics* 109, no. 1 (2002): 45–60.

Ozer, E. J. "The Effects of School Gardens on Students and Schools: Conceptualization and Considerations for Maximizing Healthy Development." *Health Education & Behavior* 34, no. 6 (2007): 846–863.

Painter, J., J. H. Rah, and Y. K. Lee. "Comparison of International Food Guide Pictorial Representations." *Journal of the American Dietetic Association* 102, no. 4 (2002): 483–489.

Plourde, G. "Preventing and Managing Pediatric Obesity. Recommendations for Family Physicians." *Canadian Family Physician* 52 (2006): 322–328.

Rigby, N. "Obesity Experts Back Junk Food Marketing Ban." International Association for the Study of Obesity/International Obesity TaskForce; 2008. [Online information; retrieved 8/8/08.] http://www.iotf.org/IASOmarketingreleaseMarch1508.htm.

Robinson, T. N. "Television Viewing and Childhood Obesity." *Pediatric Clinics of North America* 48, no. 4 (2001): 1017–1025.

St-Onge, M. P., K. L. Keller, and S. B. Heymsfield. "Changes in Child-hood Food Consumption Patterns: A Cause for Concern in Light of Increasing Body Weights." *American Journal of Clinical Nutrition* 78, no. 6 (2003): 1068–1073.

Subramanian, S. V., and G. D. Smith. "Patterns, Distribution, and Determinants of Under- and Overnutrition: A Population-based Study of Women in India." *American Journal of Clinical Nutrition* 84, no. 3 (2006): 633–640.

Summerbell, C. D., E. Waters, L. D. Edmunds, S. Kelly, T. Brown, and K. J. Campbell. "Interventions for Preventing Obesity in Children." *Cochrane Database of Systematic Reviews* 3 (2005): CD001871.

U.S. Department of Agriculture (USDA). *Dietary Guidelines for Americans, 2005.* 2005. [Online information; retrieved 1/8/09.] http://www.health.gov/dietaryguidelines/dga2005/document/.

WeCan! "Helpful Ways to Reduce Screen Time." 2008. [Online information; retrieved 1/8/09.] http://www.nhlbi.nih.gov/health/public/heart/obesity/wecan/live-it/screen-time.htm.

Weight-control Information Network (WIN). "Helping Your Overweight Child." 2008. [Online information; retrieved 1/8/09.] http://www.win.niddk.nih.gov/publications/over_child.htm.

Whitaker, R. C., J. A. Wright, M. S. Pepe, K. D. Seidel, and W. H. Dietz. "Predicting Obesity in Young Adulthood from Childhood and Parental Obesity." *New England Journal of Medicine* 337, no. 13 (1997): 869–873.

World Health Organization (WHO). "Global Strategy on Diet, Physical Activity and Health: Obesity and Overweight." Geneva: WHO, 2003.

World Health Organization (WHO). "World Health Organization Ministerial Conference on Counteracting Obesity." Copenhagen, Denmark: WHO Regional Office for Europe, 2006.

World Health Organization (WHO). "Obesity and Overweight." In *Global Strategy on Diet, Physical Activity and Health.* Geneva: WHO, 2008.

Xanthakos, S. A., S. R. Daniels, and T. H. Inge. "Bariatric Surgery in Adolescents: An Update." *Adolescent Medicine Clinics* 17, no. 3 (2006): 589–612; abstract x.

Yanovski, J. A. "Intensive Therapies for Pediatric Obesity." *Pediatric Clinics of North America* 48, no. 4 (2001): 1041–1053

4

Chronology

1942   Louis Dublin, a statistician at Metropolitan Life Insurance Company (MLIC), groups about 4 million people who were insured with Metropolitan Life into categories based on their height, body frame (small, medium, or large), and weight. People who maintained their body weight at the average for 25-year-olds are found to live the longest. As insurance companies look for criteria by which to judge the desirability of applicants, these figures become the acceptable height-weight ranges for men and women and are called "ideal weights" (MLIC 1942).

1943   Enough of the U.S. population is above ideal body weight (IBW) that the MLIC declares, "Overweight is so common that it constitutes a national health problem of the first order" (MLIC 1943).

1951   Tillie Lewis starts a new food company based in Stockton, California, that offers new low-calorie products. Lewis becomes one of the earliest marketers of diet foods with her Tasti-Diet line of artificially sweetened fruits, soft drinks, puddings, jellies, and chocolate sauce.

1952   Dr. Lester Breslow popularizes idea of optimum weight for health. In a classic paper, Breslow notes that

1952
(*cont.*)
"One out of six well people ... are 20 percent or more overweight" and that "Weight control is a major public health problem" (Breslow 1952).

1954
The first bariatric surgery is performed for which documentation is submitted to a peer-reviewed journal. Dr. Arnold Kremen and Dr. John Linner at the University of Minnesota, while studying nutrition absorption in dogs, discover that the dogs lost weight after undergoing operations that bypassed much of their intestines. In Dr. Linner's private surgical practice, one of his patients asks him to use the technique on her in the hope that she, too, will lose weight. With the successful results of that procedure, bariatric surgery is born.

1956
President Dwight Eisenhower establishes the President's Council on Physical Fitness and Sports out of concern that Americans are becoming less active. The program is a partnership between the public, private, and nonprofit sectors of society. The spark to develop the Council comes from John Kelly, who was better known as the father of actress Grace Kelly. John Kelly, a wartime physical fitness officer, believes that the current affluent lifestyle makes life so easy and effortless that adults and children are rapidly losing muscle tone.

Jack LaLanne brings his fitness and diet television program into living rooms throughout the United States. His popular television series, *The Jack LaLanne Show,* encourages viewers to get up from the chair and work out. LaLanne's belief that daily, vigorous, systematic exercise and proper diet are keys to good health is an idea supported by medical professionals in future years.

1959
The MLIC replaces the term "ideal weight" with "desirable weight" (MLIC 1959) when it is discovered that these weights are associated with the lowest mortality among people from the United States and

Canada who purchased life insurance policies from 1935 to 1954.

1960   Metrecal, a diet drink in a can, is introduced by the Mead Johnson Company as a weight-loss aid. Metrecal, taken as directed, is a complete low-calorie meal that does not require calorie counting or food preparation. It is the first in a long line of successfully promoted liquid diets that will include products such as SlimFast beverages.

1963   Jean Nidetch, a housewife from Queens, New York, starts the Weight Watchers Club, basing it on a plan that helped her lose more than 50 pounds. She invites her friends over weekly to discuss how to lose weight. The club is successful because it provides motivation, mutual support, and encouragement from people who are all working on weight loss or maintenance. Members can even become meeting leaders and share the story of their personal success with others. This enterprise will grow into Weight Watchers International, a successful business with 1 million members in groups all over the world.

1964   Dr. G. J. Hamwi develops a simple way to estimate ideal body weight. His formulas for IBW will be a popular method used in clinical practice for decades to come.

1967   Surgeon Edward E. Mason at the University of Iowa develops the first gastric bypass surgery for weight loss. Previous to this version, surgeons would just remove part of the intestine, a procedure called intestinal bypass, to reduce the number of calories the body could absorb. For a further reduction in food intake, Dr. Mason uses staples to create a small pouch in the top of the stomach. Patients would feel full eating less because there was not much room for food.

1970s   Jaw wiring is used for weight loss. This orthodontic procedure prevents the mouth from opening more

1970s   than a few centimeters. As a form of weight control, it
(*cont.*) prevents consumption of solid food, thus causing a
         reduction in calorie intake. It is suggested as a method
         to be tried before surgery is attempted.

         U.S. child obesity is estimated at 4 percent of the U.S.
         population.

1972   *Dr. Atkins' Diet Revolution* is published. Dr. Robert
         Atkins, a cardiologist, recommends eating a diet high
         in protein and fat and low in carbohydrates. He devel-
         ops the plan as a way to reduce his own overweight
         and claims that, by eating meat, fish, eggs, and cheese
         and avoiding sugars and starches, anyone can lose
         weight without counting calories. He believes this diet
         will cause excess body fat to be burned for fuel and
         will combat heart disease and diabetes. Although the
         book is a best seller, the Atkins diet is not recom-
         mended by conventional physicians and nutritionists
         because it does not follow traditional nutrition
         guidelines.

1974   The first International Congress on Obesity is held in
         London. There are 500 attendees from 30 countries.
         This meeting is organized in recognition of the need
         for continuing international assemblies of obesity
         experts and policy makers. Researchers present their
         latest findings by posting abstracts and by speaking at
         invited lectures and symposia, demonstrating the need
         for the *International Journal of Obesity,* a new journal
         devoted to global work in the field of obesity.

1980s   Body mass index (BMI) becomes an international stan-
         dard for obesity measurement.

         Liposuction is introduced in the United States. This
         procedure of removing localized fatty deposits and
         body contouring is revolutionized in 1985 when
         Dr. Jeffrey A. Klein develops a technique which per-
         mits liposuction using only local anesthesia and
         requires small incisions and little blood loss. Procedure

guidelines for this new, safer form of liposuction are approved by the American Academy of Dermatology in 1989, and numerous postgraduate courses help dermatologists learn this technique to meet a growing demand for what will become the most requested cosmetic surgery procedure.

1982   The first nonprofit professional organization to study obesity is established. The Obesity Society is committed to encouraging research on the causes and treatment of obesity and to keeping the medical community and public informed of new advances.

1983   The MLIC height-weight tables are revised again when it is discovered that the weights associated with longevity were higher than in the previous tables. Depending on height, the new tables increase the desirable weight 2 to 13 pounds for men and 3 to 8 pounds for women.

1984   The 7-Eleven convenience store outlets introduce a new size of soda—the 44-ounce Super Big Gulp.

Dr. Michael Weintraub's research on obese patients shows that a combination of two drugs, phentermine and fenfluramine (later known as fen-phen), are more effective at producing weight loss than either of the drugs alone, and in lower dosages with fewer side effects. Fenfluramine has been used for decades as a U.S. Food and Drug Administration (FDA)–approved weight loss medication, but the combination is not yet sanctioned by the FDA.

1985   The National Institutes of Health (NIH) classifies obesity as a disease. Formerly, obesity was thought to result from the single adverse behavior of eating inappropriate quantities. Studies that show that specific biochemical alterations occur in humans and experimental animals in response to environmental food and activity factors indicate that obesity meets the definition of a disease.

1985 to 1998	BMI risk categories for Americans are defined. Between 1985 and 1998, the definition of overweight in U.S. government publications is a BMI of at least 27.3 for women and 27.8 for men.
1988	The 7-Eleven stores introduce the giant 64-ounce Double Big Gulp. There are nearly 800 calories in the biggest soft drink on the market.
1989	A research study by Wadden and others shows that 98 percent of dieters regain all lost weight within five years (Wadden et al. 1989).
1990s	Leptin is discovered by several groups during this decade studying obese mice that carry a gene that makes them unable to produce any leptin. The hormone regulates energy expenditure and food intake in rodents. In response to increased fat storage, leptin is released into the bloodstream and signals to the brain that the body has had enough to eat. If no leptin is available, severe obesity occurs. When leptin is given to the animals, they decrease food intake and body weight. Although thousands of mice may be leptin deficient, fewer than 10 people in the world are obese because of absolute leptin deficiency.
1990	The Nutrition Labeling and Education Act is signed into law. This act is a new mandate for food manufacturers to provide a label with nutrient and calorie content for their products.
1991	An NIH panel endorses bypass surgery for obesity. A panel of experts from NIH reviews studies and results of surgical treatments for severely overweight individuals. It concludes that surgical alterations of the digestive system seem to work for many people without severe side effects. They approve bariatric surgery as an effective option for severely obese people who have failed more moderate weight-reduction strategies.

The National Heart, Lung and Blood Institute (NHLBI) establishes the Obesity Education Initiative to aid in decreasing the incidence of cardiovascular disease and type 2 diabetes by reducing the prevalence of over-weight and increasing physical activity in Americans.

1992   *Dr. Atkins' New Diet Revolution* is published. This updated version of Dr. Atkins' diet becomes very popular, and his company, Atkins Nutritionals, will eventually have revenues that reach $100 million a year.

The diet drug combination fen-phen is marketed aggressively as a magic weight-loss pill. Hundreds of clinics open specifically to prescribe this weight-loss medication. The number of prescriptions written for fen-phen grows from 60,000 in 1992 to 18 million in 1996. The drugs are sold under a variety of trade and generic names, including Pondimin, Fastin, Lonamin, Redux, and Adipex-P.

1993   In the first decision of its kind, a federal court of appeals panel rules that job discrimination against severely obese people violates federal disability laws. The defendant in the case maintains that she is not dis-abled by her weight; however, under the law, discrimi-nation based even on a perceived disability is illegal.

The FDA and the U.S. Department of Agriculture (USDA) issue new regulations that specify the table format and content required for nutrition labels on most foods, now including processed meat and poul-try products.

The National Weight Control Registry (NWCR) is founded at the University of Colorado by Dr. James Hill and Dr. Rena Wing. The NWCR is a long-term study of individuals 18 years and older who have suc-cessfully maintained at least a 30-pound weight loss for a year or more. About half of the participants say

1993   they lost weight on their own without any type of for-
(*cont.*) mal program.

1995   *Weighing the Options: Criteria for Evaluating Weight-
Management Programs* is published by the Institute of
Medicine (IOM) of the National Academies. The report
gives detailed guidance on how the weight-loss industry can improve its programs to help people be more
successful at long-term weight loss. It also provides
tips for consumers on selecting a reliable program that
will improve their chances of keeping lost weight off.

The International Obesity Taskforce (IOTF) is established by Dr. W. P. T. James. A major concern of IOTF
is reversing the increase in childhood obesity around
the world.

The World Health Organization (WHO) recommends a
classification for three grades of overweight using BMI
cutoff points of 25, 30, and 40. IOTF suggests an additional cutoff point of 35.

1996   The FDA approves the fat substitute olestra for use in
potato and corn chips and crackers. Because it passes
through the body unabsorbed, olestra is a zero-calorie
fat substitute. As part of the approval, the FDA
requires manufacturers to label all products made with
olestra with a statement informing consumers that
olestra may cause abdominal cramping and loose
stools in some individuals and that it reduces absorption of vitamins A, D, E, and K. These vitamins must
be added to products with olestra to compensate for
olestra's effects on these nutrients. Procter & Gamble
sells products containing Olean, a brand name for olestra. Procter & Gamble will conduct studies to monitor
olestra's long-term effects, and the FDA will formally
review the studies within 30 months (HHS 1996).

The first snack foods made with Olean are introduced
by Frito-Lay in Iowa, Wisconsin, and Colorado. The
foods are so popular that a store in Cedar Rapids,

Iowa, takes mail orders from snack lovers all across the country.

1997   A fen-phen link to heart valve damage is established when the Mayo Clinic reports 24 cases of heart valve disease in people who use the diet medication. The 24 women, who have no previous history of cardiovascular disease, show severe deformities and a buildup of a plaque-like substance on the valves of their heart that prevent them from sealing properly. This type of valve damage is a silent condition, causing no symptoms until the deterioration becomes life threatening and requires surgery to repair. More investigation shows that 271 of 291 patients who had taken fen-phen have abnormal electrocardiograms. On September 15, with growing evidence linking the drugs to potentially fatal heart and lung disorders, the manufacturer, American Home Products, removes the drug from the market.

In November 1997, a few months after the withdrawal of fen-phen, the FDA approves Meridia, a drug that falls into the same class of many antidepressants such as Prozac. It is marketed as an alternative to fen-phen.

The FDA approves orlistat (brand name Xenical) as a prescription medication to help people lose weight, and Hoffmann–La Roche Inc. releases it onto the market. Orlistat is in a group of weight-loss pills called lipase inhibitors, which act in the gastrointestinal tract to block the absorption of fat by inhibiting pancreatic enzymes. Orlistat blocks about 30 percent of ingested fat from being absorbed. Unlike other diet pills, it does not interfere in any way with brain chemistry.

1998   An expert panel convened by NIH releases a report that defines overweight as a BMI between 25 and 29.9, and obesity as a BMI of 30 or greater. These definitions will become widely used by the federal government and the broader medical and scientific communities. The cutoff points are based on evidence that health

1998
(*cont.*)
risks increase more steeply in individuals with a BMI of 25 or greater. The public begins to learn about the switch from height-weight tables to BMI as a health risk indicator when the government launches an initiative to encourage healthy eating and exercise.

The NHLBI's *Clinical Guidelines on the Identification, Evaluation, and Treatment of Overweight and Obesity in Adults* is published and distributed to primary care physicians and other health care professionals so they can begin using the new guidelines to treat their obese patients. The report lays out a new approach for assessing overweight and obesity, and it establishes evidence-based principles for safe and effective weight loss for the first time. The guidelines also provide practical strategies for implementing the recommendations.

1999
Studies show that leptin is not effective for human weight loss. The discovery of the fat-regulating hormone created great excitement when it was believed that injecting obese patients with it could produce easy weight loss. The hope among scientists and obese people is dashed when clinical trials in humans show that the hormone is not effective, as only a small amount of weight is lost, even with high doses of leptin.

Singer Carnie Wilson makes her gastric bypass surgery a public event and allows the procedure to be viewed by more than 500,000 people as it is broadcast live over the Internet. The 31-year-old woman weighed more than 300 pounds before the procedure, which reduced her stomach to the size of an egg.

Each American consumes an average of 155 pounds of caloric sweeteners (sugars, honey, corn syrups) that amount to more than 50 teaspoonfuls of added sugars per person per day.

In one year, Jared Fogle's weight decreases from 425 to 190 pounds as a result of his eating low-fat sandwiches from the Subway food outlet (Subway 2008). The

22-year-old, 6 foot, 2 inch, Indiana University student says he created a 1,000-calorie-a-day Subway diet consisting of little more than Subway sandwiches for a year. Contradicting bad press that has convinced many consumers that it is virtually impossible to lose weight while eating convenience foods, Jared proves that a low-fat, calorie-conscious, convenient diet can work.

2000   A historical moment occurs when the estimated number of overweight people in the world exceeds the number of those who are underweight.

In January, the U.S. Department of Health and Human Services (HHS) launches Healthy People 2010, a comprehensive, nationwide health promotion and disease prevention agenda. The plan is designed to be a framework for improving the health of all people in the United States during the first decade of the 21st century. The promotion builds upon previous initiatives that had been proposed over the preceding two decades. The goals of increasing quality and years of healthy life and elimination of health disparities are broken down into objectives that will be used to measure progress. Each objective has a target to be achieved by 2010.

The IOTF Childhood Obesity Working Group publishes standard definitions for overweight and obesity in childhood. Prior to its publication, agreement has been lacking about the definition of overweight and obesity in childhood and adolescence, with only arbitrary cutoff points being used to identify childhood obesity.

Based on the Behavioral Risk Factor Surveilance System, 46 percent of U.S. women and 33 percent of U.S. men said they were trying to lose weight. (C. L. Bish, 2005).

2001   In the "Surgeon General's Call to Action to Prevent and Decrease Overweight and Obesity 2001," U.S. Surgeon General David Satcher declares obesity to be a

2001
(*cont.*) public health epidemic that could be the cause of as much preventable disease and death as cigarette smoking. He says, "Health problems resulting from overweight and obesity could reverse many of the health gains achieved in the U.S. in recent decades" (HHS 2001). This call to action is intended to promote the recognition of obesity as a health problem and to develop programs to treat obesity and encourage people to change their eating and exercise habits.

2002 The Federal Trade Commission (FTC) releases a report titled *Weight Loss Advertising: An Analysis of Current Trends*, indicating that the use of false and misleading claims in weight-loss advertising is widespread. Researchers examine 300 weight-loss advertisements taken from television, radio, the Internet, newspapers, magazines, e-mail, and direct mail. They find that 55 percent of weight-loss ads make claims that are misleading, lack proof, or are obviously false. Although the FTC study does not criticize specific products, it provides examples of false or exaggerated claims and warns that some weight-loss supplements lack safety warnings and can be dangerous.

Obesity treatment gets a boost when the Internal Revenue Service recognizes obesity as a disease and allows payments for medically valid obesity treatments to be claimed as a medical tax deduction.

2003 The FTC launches a campaign to educate U.S. media outlets about false weight-loss claims. The promotion, called the Red Flag Campaign, is an attempt to expose advertisements that are fraudulent and scientifically impossible. The FTC report, based on a 2002 Weight-Loss Advertising Workshop, concludes that the claims are not scientifically feasible at the current time for nonprescription drugs, dietary supplements, creams, wraps, and patches. The FTC produces a reference guide so that media outlets can screen out bogus claims by checking through the list without having to go into in-depth investigations on their own.

At a congressional briefing in 2003, Surgeon General Richard H. Carmona declares that obesity is an epidemic as he speaks about the "obesity crisis in America." He calls obesity a health crisis that is the fastest-growing cause of disease and death in the United States (Carmona 2003). Nearly two out of every three Americans are overweight or obese. One out of every eight deaths in the United States is caused by an illness directly related to overweight and obesity.

In the first-ever policy statement exclusively focused on identifying and preventing childhood obesity, the American Academy of Pediatrics asks pediatricians to go beyond their routine tracking of height and weight. The group wants doctors to use the body mass index for children and adolescents. The policy instructs pediatricians to promote healthy eating patterns and physical activity at each office visit.

In the United States, young people spend an average of almost 6.5 hours a day with electronic media such as televisions, radios, video players, and computers. That figure represents an increase of more than an hour since 2000.

The FDA eliminates the warning label on snack foods containing olestra fat replacers that the agency had required since 1996. After reviewing studies submitted by Proctor & Gamble as well as adverse event reports submitted by the Center for Science in the Public Interest, the FDA concluded that the label statement was no longer warranted. Studies of consumers who ate products containing olestra showed olestra caused only mild gastrointestinal consequences, effects that also occurred with consumption of full fat products (FDA 2003).

2004   The population obesity rate for American children ages 6 to 11 years is 19 percent, and for 12- to 19-year-old

2004
(*cont.*)
adolescents, the rate is 17 percent. Foretelling a future with more obese children and adolescents, data this year show that more than 10 percent of younger children (ages two to five) are overweight. That percentage is up from 7 percent in 1994.

The *Strategic Plan for NIH Obesity Research* is released. The NIH Research Task Force publishes this multifaceted agenda for the study of behavioral and environmental causes of obesity along with the study of genetic and biologic causes. The plan details coordination of obesity research across NIH.

In February, the FDA bans the sale of all dietary supplements in the United States that contain ephedrine. The agency says these supplements create an unreasonable risk of illness and injury.

A controversial independent film called *Super Size Me* by Morgan Spurlock is introduced as an exploration of the prevalence of obesity in the United States. Spurlock eats only food from the McDonald's menu for a month. He starts as a healthy man, but as his experiment progresses, he becomes overweight and experiences issues with his health. This film causes McDonald's to make alterations in their menu and is followed by similar documentaries.

Research study reveals that 30 percent of children eat fast food on a daily basis. The findings suggest that fast-food consumption has increased fivefold among children since 1970.

To promote healthy lifestyles for adults and children in all countries, WHO develops the Global Strategy on Diet, Physical Activity and Health (DPAS). This program is endorsed by the 57th World Health Assembly in May 2004.

The IOTF report *Obesity in Children and Young People: A Crisis in Public Health*, alerts that childhood obesity is increasing in both developed and developing countries. The report, delivered to WHO while government ministers in Geneva are debating the adoption of the Global Strategy on Diet, Physical Activity and Health, warns that obesity significantly increases the risk that children may develop type 2 diabetes, heart disease, and a variety of adverse health consequences that may not become evident until adulthood.

McDonald's fast food outlets plan to phase out Super Size french fries and soft drinks as the world's largest restaurant chain promotes its Eat Smart, Be Active initiative. McDonald's is adding salads and moving to provide more fruit, vegetable, and yogurt options with children's Happy Meals. The new program is designed to put McDonald's into a position of being part of the solution to the obesity issue, rather than part of the problem.

2005   The 2005 *Dietary Guidelines for Americans* is released. The report gives advice on healthful food and physical activity choices for the general public older than two years of age. The basic premise of the *Dietary Guidelines* is that nutrient needs are best met through consuming foods. Each five-year revision of the guidelines is based on analysis of the latest scientific information by the Dietary Guidelines Advisory Committee and forms the basis for USDA and HHS program and policy development. Because it contains technical information, the *Dietary Guidelines* is generally more accessible to policy makers, nutrition educators, nutritionists, and health care providers than to the general public. In order for individuals to follow the guidelines in their daily life, the dietary recommendations are presented as healthy eating patterns such as the USDA Food Guide and the DASH (Dietary Approaches to Stop Hypertension) Eating Plan. The guidelines are depicted graphically as the Food Guide Pyramid, which recommends types and amounts of foods from seven food groups and daily physical activity.

2005
(*cont.*)

On April 14, a judge in a federal district court overturns the FDA ephedra ban as a result of a suit brought by the Nutraceutical Corporation, a supplement manufacturer. The judge concludes that there is not enough scientific evidence to prove that those products with 10 milligrams or less of ephedrine in a daily dose pose a health risk.

A team of experts on aging and obesity concludes that the steady rise in human life expectancy during the past two centuries may soon come to an end. The epidemic of obesity and related health risks could cause a decline in Americans' life expectancy and could cancel out the life-extending benefits of advances in medicine. Further, it predicts that young people, who are becoming obese at unprecedented rates, will experience the greatest loss of longevity. This prediction leads to the controversial idea that children today may live less healthy and shorter lives than their parents.

An IOM report, *Preventing Childhood Obesity: Health in the Balance*, offers a guide for coordinating contributions from government, schools, industry, media, and families. The plan is the most comprehensive analysis to date on the problems and potential solutions related to the childhood obesity epidemic.

2006

A federal appeals court reinstates the FDA ban on ephedra-containing supplements. The court rules that more than 19,000 adverse events reported to the FDA provide enough evidence to uphold the initial ban. The FDA declares that no dose of ephedrine in dietary supplements is safe and that sale of these products is illegal.

The southeastern region of the United States has the highest prevalence of obesity and overweight. With prevalence equal to or greater than 30 percent of their population, Mississippi and West Virginia lead all the states in number of citizens who are obese.

New York City's Department of Health and Mental Hygiene becomes the first agency to require that any restaurant chain with 15 or more nationwide outlets show calorie information on menus, menu boards, and food tags. That directive includes about 10 percent of the restaurants in the five boroughs of New York City—Manhattan, Brooklyn, Queens, the Bronx, and Staten Island. Advocates of similar menu-labeling measures say this requirement paves the way for other local and state governments to pass such ordinances.

The Robert Wood Johnson Foundation requests that IOM have an expert committee examine the progress that had been made in preventing childhood obesity in the United States. The resulting report, *Progress in Preventing Childhood Obesity: How Do We Measure Up?* presents specific actions for childhood obesity prevention. Lack of a system for monitoring progress was identified as a stumbling block to evaluating ongoing programs. The committee encouraged continuing surveillance and assessment systems to track effectiveness of existing nutrition programs.

2007   An over-the-counter version of the prescription weight-loss drug orlistat is approved by the FDA. This approval marks the first time that the FDA has found an over-the-counter weight-loss product to actually work. The drug, sold under the brand name Alli, is a reduced-strength version of Xenical and works in the same way, decreasing absorption of fat in the intestines. In addition to using the drug, Alli purchasers are encouraged to follow an online diet plan that includes menus and shopping lists and to join a network of other Alli users who provide support.

The AMA begins a campaign to educate physicians about how to prevent and manage childhood obesity.

2007   The goal is to introduce obesity training as part of
(*cont.*)   undergraduate, graduate, and continuing medical
           education programs. The committee creates 22 recom-
           mendations for health care professionals who provide
           obesity care to apply in their practices.

           Progress toward coordinating the work of the federal
           and state governments' existing childhood obesity pre-
           vention programs was made when HHS created the
           Childhood Overweight and Obesity Prevention Initia-
           tive. The Initiative encourages community-based inter-
           ventions, such as the NIH We Can! (Ways to Enhance
           Children's Activity and Nutrition) program; the Presi-
           dent's Council on Physical Fitness and Sports'
           National Fitness Challenge; and the National Center
           for Physical Development and Outdoor Play, which
           will help improve outdoor play for children in Head
           Start programs.

           The National Center on Health Statistics report *Obesity
           among Adults in the United States—No Change since
           2003–2004* is the latest analysis based on the National
           Health and Nutrition Examination Survey data. Its
           contents may represent the first sign that the obesity
           epidemic could be peaking as a result of prevention
           and management programs sponsored by the
           government and health care organizations and by indi-
           viduals' personal effort to control weight. Although
           the obesity prevalence at this time has not measurably
           increased in the past few years, levels are still high.
           More than one-third of adults (more than 72 million
           people) were obese in 2005–2006. This figure includes
           33.3 percent of men and 35.3 percent of women. These
           percentages are not statistically different from 2003–
           2004, when 31.1 percent of men and 33.2 percent of
           women were obese.

2008   At 97 years old, Jack LaLanne, known as the godfather
           of the American fitness movement, is inducted into the

California Hall of Fame by California first lady Maria Shriver.

In a progress review of the Healthy People 2010 (HP 2010) government initiative, representatives from the FDA and NIH examine its objectives to promote healthy weights among children and adolescents and healthy eating among all Americans. Three targets are directly related to obesity.

The first target is to increase the proportion of adults who are at a healthy weight to 60 percent of Americans. The review shows that the proportion of adults whose weight is in the healthy range was 32 percent during 2003–2006, a decrease from 42 percent in the years 1988–1994.

The second target is to reduce the proportion of adults who are obese to 15 percent or less of the population. In the review period, 33 percent of adults were obese in 2003–2006 compared with a 1988–1994 baseline of 23 percent.

The third goal is to reduce the proportion of children and adolescents who are overweight or obese. The target for both children and adolescents is 5 percent. Overweight and obesity in children and adolescents increased from 11 percent in 1988–1994 to about 17 percent in 2003–2006. Although data indicate that yearly increases in overweight and obesity are slowing or reaching a plateau, the number of people who have an unhealthy weight remains unacceptably high. The conclusion that can be drawn from this examination is that, in 2008, Americans have made little progress toward the HP 2010 targets.

In collaboration with the Robert Wood Johnson Foundation, IOM establishes the Standing Committee on Childhood Obesity Prevention. The committee will aid in integrating ideas and programs from government, academia, and corporate sectors and will report

2008   on the most promising solutions to preventing child-
(*cont.*)   hood obesity. It will continue to monitor progress
           toward implementing the recommendations of its first
           report on preventing childhood obesity, released in
           2005.

References

Bish, C. L. "Diet and Physical Activity Behaviors among Americans Trying to Lose Weight: 2000 Behavioral Risk Factor Surveillance System." *Obesity Research* 13, no. 3 (2005): 596–607.

Breslow, L. "Public Health Aspects of Weight Control." *American Journal of Public Health and the Nation's Health* 42, no. 9 (1952): 1116–1120.

Carmona, R. "The Obesity Crisis in America." In *Testimony before the Subcommittee on Education Reform Committee on Education and the Workforce United States House of Representatives,* edited by Surgeon General, U.S. Public Health Service. Washington, DC: U.S. Department of Health and Human Services, 2003.

Metropolitan Life Insurance Company (MLIC). "Metropolitan Life Insurance Company. Ideal Weights for Men 1942." *Statistical Bulletin—Metropolitan Life Insurance Company* 23 (1942): 6–8.

Metropolitan Life Insurance Company (MLIC). "Metropolitan Life Insurance Company. Ideal Weights for Women." *Statistical Bulletin—Metropolitan Life Insurance Company* 24 (1943): 6–8.

Metropolitan Life Insurance Company (MLIC). "New Weight Standards for Men and Women." *Statistical Bulletin—Metropolitan Life Insurance Company* 40 (1959): 1–10.

Subway Restaurants. "All about Jared." 2008. http://www.subway.com/subwayroot/menunutrition/jared/jaredsStory.aspx.

U.S. Department of Health and Human Services (HHS). "FDA Approves Fat Substitute, Olestra." 1996. [Online press release; retrieved 1/8/09.] http://www.fda.gov/bbs/topics/NEWS/NEW00524.html.

U.S. Department of Health and Human Services (HHS). "The Surgeon General's Call to Action to Prevent and Decrease Overweight and Obesity." 2001. [Online information; retrieved 1/8/09.] http://

www.surgeongeneral.gov/topics/obesity/calltoaction/Callto
Action.pdf.

U.S. Food and Drug Administration (FDA). "FDA Changes Labeling
Requirement for Olestra." 2003. [Online information; retrieved 1/8/
09.] http://www.fda.gov/bbs/topics/ANSWERS/2003/ANS01245
.html.

Wadden, T. A., J. A. Sternberg, K. A. Letizia, A. J. Stunkard, and G. D.
Foster. "Treatment of Obesity by Very Low Calorie Diet, Behavior
Therapy, and Their Combination: A Five-Year Perspective."
International Journal of Obesity 13, Suppl. 2 (1989): 39–46.

5

Biographical Sketches

This chapter presents short biographies of more than 50 people who are important in the topic of obesity. The subjects of these biographies include researchers, policy makers, people visible in the media, and those who promote certain diet/exercise programs. The biographies range from businessperson Jean Nidetch, founder of Weight Watchers, to Jack LaLanne, known as the godfather of fitness, to public personalities such as TV's Oprah Winfrey, who has battled obesity for many years, and Jared Fogle, the man who lost 250 pounds by eating Subway sandwiches.

The chapter also highlights researchers such as Dr. Ethan Sims, who coined the word "diabesity" to refer to obesity-induced type 2 diabetes. This section also highlights people who are considered to be controversial in the weight-management field, such as Dr. Robert Atkins, who developed the Atkins diet, which is high in protein and fat and low in carbohydrates, and Dr. Dean Ornish, who developed a high complex carbohydrate diet that is low in fat.

Obesity is a global epidemic but the vast majority of the people listed are from the United States. In addition, many more men than women are profiled. At this time, more women are entering this field, and many of them will likely be notable "movers and shakers" in the future.

S. Daniel Abraham (1924–)

S. Daniel Abraham was born and raised in Long Beach, New York. He served as an infantryman in the U.S. Army during

World War II. After the war, he bought a small pharmaceutical company, Thompson Medical. In the late 1950s, he introduced his first diet product, Slim-Mint gum, which contained benzocaine and was supposed to decrease hunger. This was followed in 1976 by Dexatrim, which was a one-a-day weight-loss pill that contained phenylpropanolamine (PPA). It was reformulated when PPA was linked to an increased risk of strokes. The "new" Dexatrim contained ephedrine, which was linked to adverse health effects, and Dexatrim was reformulated again.

In the late 1970s, Abraham "shook up the weight-loss industry" by producing the nutrition drink Slim-Fast, according to *Forbes*. The drink made losing weight simpler. He sold the company to Unilever for $2.3 billion in 2000.

David Allison (1963–)

David Allison was born in New York City. He has a BA (Vassar College, 1985) and a PhD (Hofstra University, 1990). He was a researcher at New York Obesity Research Center from 1991 to 1994 and held assistant and associate professor posts at Columbia University College of Physicians and Surgeons from 1994 to 2001. In 2001, he became professor of biostatistics, head of the Section on Statistical Genetics, and director of the National Institutes of Health (NIH)–funded Clinical Nutrition Research at University of Alabama, Birmingham.

Allison's research casts a wide net. He is particularly known for his work on the relations among obesity, weight loss, and mortality or longevity and for his work on the genetic and environmental influences on obesity. He is also known for challenging conventional ideas, exploring novel hypotheses, and holding himself and others to rigorous standards of evidence. He has authored more than 300 scientific papers and edited five books. Allison has received a number of awards, including the Lilly Scientific Achievement Award (Obesity Society, 2002) and the Andre Mayer Award (International Association for the Study of Obesity [IASO], 2002). He received the Presidential Award for Excellence in Science, Mathematics and Engineering Mentoring (2006) and met with President George W. Bush in the Oval Office.

When asked about his work, he responded, "Science is a wonderful calling—a true vocation. I can imagine no better walk of life than surrounding oneself with bright colleagues, exchanging ideas and pursuing unanswered questions" (Allison, pers. comm.).

Arne Astrup (1955–)

Arne Astrup was born in Frederiksberg, Denmark. He obtained his degrees in medicine (1981) and doctorate (1986) from the Faculty of Health Sciences, University of Copenhagen. Astrup is professor and head of the Department of Human Nutrition at the Royal Veterinary and Agriculture University of Copenhagen. Some of his research investigates a newly discovered hormone, adiponectin, which is thought to improve insulin sensitivity and to decrease the risk of development of atherosclerosis. Weight loss increases plasma adiponectin, which is a hormone secreted by adipose tissue.

Astrup is internationally known for his leadership in the field of obesity. He is president of the International Association for the Study of Obesity (2006–2010) and editor in chief of *Obesity Reviews* (1999–). Some of his many awards include Knight of the Order of Danneborg (1999), Servier Award for Outstanding Obesity Research (1999), and IASO Andre Mayer Award (1994).

Robert C. Atkins (1930–2003)

Robert C. Atkins was born in Columbus, Ohio. He received his BA from the University of Michigan in 1951 and his MD from Cornell Medical College in 1955. He was a physician and cardiologist and the founder of the Atkins Center for Complementary Medicine. In 1963, he was gaining a lot of weight and came upon an article in the *Journal of the American Medical Association* stating that one does not have to go on a low-calorie diet to lose weight but can choose a low-carbohydrate diet instead. He subsequently built his diet around eating meat, shrimp, duck, and fish and very little carbohydrates. As a result, he lost a lot of weight easily. In a 2003 interview by Larry King on CNN, Atkins was introduced as being "the world's most controversial diet guru."

Atkins is best known for his popular diet, which features very low intake of carbohydrates and high intake of protein and fat. His diet allows steak, eggs, and cheese, but not chocolate. His first diet book, *Dr. Atkins' Diet Revolution: The High Calorie Way to Stay Thin Forever*, was published in 1972. The Atkins diet plan has since been modified to include more carbohydrates, which are gradually introduced after about a week, whereas it severely restricts refined carbohydrates to less than 50 calories daily, or about 1 tablespoon of sugar. His books have appeared in the number one spot on the *New York Times* best-seller lists.

A number of celebrities adopted the Atkins diet, including Julia Roberts, Catherine Zeta-Jones, Brad Pitt, and Al Gore. Stevie Nicks, of Fleetwood Mac, called Atkins "a God among men." He died in 2003 from injuries sustained by slipping on ice. The headline for his obituary in *The Guardian* read, "Diet guru who grew fat on the proceeds of the carbohydrate revolution" (Leith, 2003).

Richard L. Atkinson (1942–)

Richard L. Atkinson was born in Petersburg, Virginia. He graduated from Virginia Military Institute (1964) and received his MD from the Medical College of Virginia (1968). He was a faculty member at the University of Virginia (1977–1983), University of California, Davis (1983–1987), Eastern Virginia Medical School (1987–1993), and University of Wisconsin (1993–2002).

Atkinson is known for his pioneering research in virus-induced obesity. Atkinson and his colleague Dr. Nikhil Dhurandhar demonstrated that a human adenovirus (Ad-36) produces obesity in animals and is associated with obesity in humans. Their research was not initially accepted by the scientific community; in fact, it was dismissed and heavily criticized. Today, their research is viewed as an important breakthrough that may help to explain our worldwide obesity epidemic.

Atkinson also conducted some of the early research on intestinal bypass surgery. His wife, Susan, learned about surgery in her father's laboratory, and she then taught Atkinson to perform surgery on obese rats.

Atkinson is editor of the *International Journal of Obesity* (2000–). He is clinical professor of pathology at Virginia Commonwealth University and director of the Obetach Obesity Research Center. Atkinson and Dr. Judith S. Stern are cofounders of the American Obesity Association (1995), a lay advocacy organization that is now part of The Obesity Society (TOS). Atkinson and Stern were the first recipients, in 2006, of the Atkinson-Stern Award for Distinguished Public Service, awarded annually by The Obesity Society.

George Blackburn (1936–)

George Blackburn was born in McPherson, Kansas. He has an MD (University of Kansas, 1965) and a PhD in nutritional biochemistry (Massachusetts Institute of Technology, 1973). He pioneered the development of the Roux-en-Y bypass operation for weight loss in very obese people.

Blackburn is the S. Daniel Abraham Associate Professor of Surgery and Nutrition, associate director of the Nutrition Division at Harvard Medical School, and director of the Center for Nutrition Medicine at Beth Israel Deaconess Medical Center. He is committed to expanding research and treatment for obesity and nutrition. Blackburn was past president of The Obesity Society, American Society for Clinical Nutrition, and American Society of Parenteral Nutrition. He cochairs the Reality Coalition, an organization aiming to promote healthy, moderate weight loss.

Blackburn has published more than 400 papers. Some of his honors are the Grace Goldsmith Award (American College of Nutrition, 1988) and Goldberger Award in Clinical Nutrition (American Medical Association, 1998). He is an honorary member of the American Dietetic Association (1992). He says of his life and studies, "I want to leave the world better off than when I received it" (Blackburn, pers. comm.).

Steven N. Blair (1939–)

Steven N. Blair was born in Mankato, Kansas. He received his BA from Kansas Wesleyan University in 1962 and his PED in physical education from Indiana University. In 1966, he became physical education instructor at the University of South Carolina and progressed through the ranks to professor. He worked at the Dallas-based Cooper Institute for 22 years, where he was first a researcher, then director of research, and ultimately president and chief executive officer. Blair returned to the University of South Carolina in 2006 as professor.

He studies the associations between lifestyle and health, with a specific emphasis on exercise, physical fitness, body composition, and chronic disease. He found that American seniors who get a regular dose of physical activity live longer than unfit adults, regardless of their measure of body fat. He has published more than 410 papers and chapters and served as senior scientific editor for the *U.S. Surgeon General's Report on Physical Activity and Health*.

According to Blair, "By 2030, approximately 70 million people will be older than 65. Nearly one-third of Americans are obese, and the majority of adults do not get enough physical activity" (Blair, pers. comm.) Medical expenditures associated with inactivity and obesity are greatest among older adults. He continues, "This is a significant economic burden to society by an aging population that is inactive and obese." Some of Blair's numerous awards and honors include three honorary doctorates, the Surgeon General's Medallion, and the Honor Award (American College of Sports Medicine).

He emphasizes that one does not have to be thin to benefit from being physically active. Thirty minutes of moderate-intensity physical activity five days per week is enough to put people in the moderate fitness category. Blair acknowledges that he is not as thin as he once was and that there is a history of obesity and heart disease in his family. However, he is physically active, having run close to 80,000 miles, and eats a healthy diet.

Claude Bouchard (1939–)

Claude Bouchard was born in Quebec, Canada. He has earned bachelor's (Laval University, 1962), master's (University of Oregon, 1963), and doctoral (University of Texas, Austin, 1977) degrees. He held the Donald Brown Research Chair on Obesity at Laval University from 1997 to 1999. Since 1999, he has served as executive director of the Pennington Biomedical Research Center in Baton Rouge, Louisiana, one of the world's leading nutrition and preventive medicine research centers.

Bouchard's most influential work is in studying the response of identical twins to long-term overfeeding. In his study, twins were overfed a total of 84,000 calories over 12 weeks.

They gained, on average, almost 15.5 pounds. Some sets of twins were low gainers and others were high gainers, but individual pairs of twins gained a similar amount of weight.

Bouchard has written several books and more than 800 scientific papers. He was president of The Obesity Society from 1991 to 1992 and the International Association for the Study of Obesity from 2002 to 2006) and was a member of the Board of the American Obesity Association. Some of his honors include the American College of Sports Medicine Citation (1992), an honorary doctorate from the Royal Academy of Medicine of Belgium, and the TOPS Award from The Obesity Society.

Bouchard is optimistic about research in obesity. However, he is pessimistic about society's ability to deal with the worldwide problem, especially with prevention of obesity. He does not foresee people changing their lifestyles so that everyone becomes physically active and adopts a prudent diet (Bouchard, pers. comm.).

George A. Bray (1931–)

George A. Bray was born in Evanston, Illinois. He has a BA from Brown University and an MD from Harvard Medical School. Bray is a leader in promoting the concept that obesity is a disease and not the result of gluttony, sloth, and moral deficit. He also has an interest in the history of medicine.

He was the first executive director of the Pennington Biomedical Research Center (1989–1998), where he is currently Boyd Professor and professor emeritus of medicine at Louisiana State University.

Bray's contributions to the field of obesity are impressive. He is recognized among his peers in the field for his research in obesity and diabetes and has published more than 1,500 scientific papers, reviews, books, and abstracts. He cofounded and was president of The Obesity Society and was founder and editor of three scientific journals. While editor of *Obesity Research* (now *Obesity*), he wrote a series of 36 historical essays that have been collected in a book called *The Battle of the Bulge* (Dorrance, 2007). He was president of the International Association for the Study of Obesity and American Society for Clinical Nutrition, and was a board member of the American Obesity Association.

Examples of his many honors include the Bristol-Myers/ Squibb Mead Johnson Award in Nutrition, Fellow of American Association for the Advancement of Science, Goldberger Award in Nutrition (American Medical Association), and Stunkard Lifetime Award (Obesity Society). The Obesity Society gives the George Bray Founder's Award in recognition of people who make significant contributions to the field that advance the clinical or scientific basis for understanding or treating obesity.

Jane E. Brody (no dates available)

Jane E. Brody is a columnist for the *New York Times*. She received her BS from Cornell University in 1962 and her MS from the University of Wisconsin School of Journalism in 1963. She joined the *New York Times* in 1965, where she specialized in medicine and biology and became the newspaper's personal health columnist in 1976. Her weekly column is syndicated in more than 100 newspapers. In one column, she wrote that the way to lose weight in 2008 is the same as it has been every other year, because the basics of good nutrition have not changed. She has appeared on numerous radio and TV shows, which earned her the title of "High Priestess of Health" from *Time* magazine (Brody, 2008).

One of her first books was *Jane Brody's Nutrition Book: A Lifetime Guide to Good Eating for Better Health and Weight Control* (Bantam, 1986). She has been awarded honorary degrees by four universities.

Brody's own diet focuses on vegetables, fruits, grains, potatoes, beans, and peas, along with low-fat dairy, fish and shellfish, lean meats, and poultry. She is active daily and walks, bikes, swims, ice skates, plays tennis, hikes, gardens, and does cross-country skiing. On her 50th birthday, Brody received a T-shirt that said, "Still Perfect—After All These Years." After she stopped laughing, she realized that it should have said, "Still Trying After All These Years" (Brody).

Kelly Brownell (1951–)

Kelly Brownell was born in Evansville, Indiana. He holds a BA in psychology from Purdue University (1973) and a PhD from

Rutgers University (1977). Brownell is professor of psychology, epidemiology, and public health, and director of the Rudd Center for Food Policy and Obesity at Yale University.

One of Brownell's famous early studies was conducted in a shopping mall, a train station, and a bus terminal in Philadelphia, where stairs and escalators were adjacent to each other. He placed a simple, colorful sign that read, "Your Heart Needs Exercise, Here's Your Chance." Brownell found that the number of people using the stairs increased following placement of the sign but that fewer obese people took the stairs.

Brownell coined the phrase "toxic environment," which applies to the many factors that have contributed to obesity. These include food marketing directed at children, large portion sizes, foods in schools, economic imbalance where healthy foods cost more than unhealthy foods, lobbying strength of food and agribusiness companies, and failure to harness the law in the service of improving nutrition. One of his books, *Food Fight* (McGraw-Hill 2003), cowritten with Katherine Battle Horgen, details these environmental drivers of obesity and proposes a number of possible policy solutions. He has applied the quote from Mohandas Gandhi about social movements to the obesity crisis: "First they ignore you. Then they laugh at you. Then they fight you. Then you win."

Brownell has written 14 books and published more than 300 scientific papers and articles. He consults with members of the U.S. Congress, appears often on television, and is frequently quoted in newspapers and magazines. In 2006, he was named by *Time* magazine as one of the World's 100 Most Influential People. One of his honors is his election to the National Academies Institute of Medicine.

Henry Buckwald (1932–)

Henry Buckwald was born in Vienna, Austria. He has an MD (Columbia University, 1957), an MS, and a PhD (University of Minnesota). He is professor in the Department of Surgery at the University of Minnesota and was holder of the Davidson Wangensteen Chair in Experimental Surgery.

Buckwald is known for his work in bariatric surgery, especially with respect to its comorbid outcomes. He has helped to improve both the type of operations done and the overall quality of bariatric surgeons. One of his seminal research studies, published 40 years ago, demonstrated that even before weight loss occurs, bariatric surgery improves insulin resistance and decreases LDL, or "bad," cholesterol.

Buckwald served as president of three organizations: the Central Surgical Association, American Society for Bariatric Surgery, and International Federation for the Surgery of Obesity. He is head of the Obesity Coalition, a national organization that includes most of the major academic groups in the United States; one of its missions involves obesity management. He also is chair of the American College of Surgeons National Faculty for Bariatric Surgery (2003–). Buckwald is a member of the Minnesota Hall of Fame (1988) in recognition of establishing the field of metabolic surgery, which later evolved into bariatric surgery.

Paul F. Campos (no date available)

Paul F. Campos is a native of Colorado. He has a bachelor's, master's, and law degree from the University of Michigan (1982, 1983, and 1989, respectively). After obtaining his JD, he worked for a Chicago law firm. In 1990, he joined the faculty at the University of Colorado Law School (Boulder), where he is now professor of law. Campos writes a regular column on political, social, and legal issues for the *Rocky Mountain News*.

Mr. Campos is the author of *The Obesity Myth: Why America's Obsession with Weight is Hazardous to Your Health* (Gotham 2004). His book is an exposé of the hysteria surrounding weight and health in U.S. society. He has questioned the association between obesity and higher mortality rates. Campos believes that the use of the body mass index (BMI) accounts for the great increase in obesity in the United States. According to Campos, if categorized using BMI, Brad Pitt is overweight and George Clooney is obese. Campos's message is that perhaps fat is not all that bad. However, some of Campos's conclusions serve to undermine the credibility of the book. For example, he concludes that "Fat Politics" played a significant role in the impeachment of President Clinton (Campos, 2004).

William J. Clinton (1946–)

William Jefferson Clinton was born in Hope, Arkansas. He served as president of the United States from 1993 to 2001. President Clinton has battled obesity all his life. Upon having quadruple bypass surgery in 2004, he decided to help prevent overweight in children. Using the resources of his foundation and teaming up with the American Heart Association, President Clinton's goal is to reduce obesity-related health problems by starting children on a lifelong path that includes proper diet and exercise. He is leading by example by cutting down on french fries, eating more fruits and vegetables, and exercising in the morning. He works with the food and restaurant industries, the media, and schools to help deliver his message. Two of his goals for schools are to have programs to increase physical activity and to improve lunches. He commented, "We've got too many kids too over-weight and they're walking time bombs" (Clinton, 2005). President Clinton received the Atkinson-Stern Award for Distinguished Public Service from The Obesity Society (2007).

Jenny Craig (1932–)

Jenny Craig was born Genevieve Guidroz in Berwick, Louisiana, and raised in New Orleans. She worked for a weight-loss company, Nutrisystem, then Craig and her husband, Sid, moved to Australia for two years, where she started the Jenny Craig Weight Loss Program in 1983 because no comprehensive weight-loss program existed in Australia at that time. She knows what it is like to be obese, having gained 50 pounds with the birth of her second daughter. Jenny Craig, Inc. has weight-loss centers in the United States, Canada, Puerto Rico, and New Zealand. In 2002, the couple sold the majority of their interests in Jenny Craig, Inc. to a New York and London–based private investment firm, ACI Capital.

William H. Dietz (no dates available)

William H. Dietz has an MD from The University of Pennsylvania (1970) and a PhD from the Massachusetts Institute of

Technology. He is one of the first researchers to pay attention to the issues surrounding overweight in children and has published more than 100 papers and is the editor of four books.

Dietz has served as the director of the Division of Nutrition and Physical Activity at the Centers for Disease Control and Prevention (CDC) since 1997. He is also a past president of the American Society of Clinical Nutrition and The Obesity Society. He helps states to develop and evaluate strategies to prevent obesity. This approach is based, in part, on Dietz's research indicating that some process takes place during adolescence that makes a person more susceptible to the complications of obesity as an adult.

Some of his honors include election to the Institute of Medicine of the National Academies (2000), recipient of the John Stalker Award (American School Food Service Association), and the George Bray Founders Award (Obesity Society, 2005).

In an interview on The Global Epidemic of Obesity, he was asked the question: What can be done about obesity? In response he encouraged adolescents to be fit, to do things with their friends, and to think about activities that are fun to do instead of watching television. Soft drinks and 10-percent juice make up 13 percent of the daily caloric intake of adolescents. Teenagers should be encouraged to drink water when they are thirsty and to start meals with soup or a salad to have less room for foods high in calories (The Global Epidemic of Obesity, 2005).

Adam Drewnowski (1948–)

Adam Drewnowski was born in Warsaw, Poland. He has a BA from Oxford University (1971) and a PhD from The Rockefeller University (1978). He is director of the Nutritional Science Program and director of the Center for Public Health Nutrition and University of Washington (Seattle) Center for obesity research.

Drewnowski's research focuses on the relationships between poverty and obesity, links between diabetes and obesity rates in vulnerable populations, and access to healthy foods. According to Drewnowski, "Energy-dense foods rich in starch, sugar or fat are the cheapest option for the consumer. As long as the healthier lean meats, fish, and fresh produce are more expensive, obesity will continue to be a problem for the working poor" (Drewnowski, pers. comm.).

Johanna Dwyer (1938–)

Johanna Dwyer was born in Syracuse, New York. She has a BS (Cornell University, 1960), an MS (University of Wisconsin, 1962), and a second MS and an ScD (Harvard University School of Public Health, 1969). She is professor of Medicine and Community Health at the School of Medicine and Freidman School of Science Nutrition and Public Policy, Tufts University, and senior nutritionist at the Office of Dietary Supplements, NIH.

Dwyer was a member of the U.S. Dietary Guidelines Committee (2000) and the Food and Nutrition Board of the National Academies (1992–2001). Her many honors include election to the National Academies Institute of Medicine (2000) and receipt of the Atwater and Elvejhem awards (American Society of Nutrition [ASN], 2005). She is a past president of ASN and the Society for Nutrition Education. She is also editor of *Nutrition Today*.

Dwyer's career has been devoted to expanding the scientific basis for clinical and public health interventions, especially in obesity and cardiovascular disease. She has published more than 475 scientific articles. Dwyer agrees with her mentor, Jean Mayer (the late president of Tufts University), that "Nutrition is not a discipline, but an agenda of problems that must be solved" (Dwyer, pers. comm.).

Katherine M. Flegal (1944–)

Katherine M. Flegal was born in Berkeley, California. She has a PhD from Cornell University (1982) and completed a postdoctoral fellowship in epidemiology at the University of Pittsburgh (1984). She was a research faculty member at the University of Michigan from 1984 to 1987 prior to joining the National Centers for Health Statistics at CDC, where she began serving in 1987.

Flegal is internationally known for her research in the epidemiology of obesity. She studies changing prevalences and epidemiologic trends of overweight in children and adults in the United States as well as causes of death. To quote Flegal, "The relation between weight and mortality is complex and varies considerably by cause of death" (Flegal, pers. comm.). She determined that BMI is not a strong predictor of death rates. People who are overweight (BMI 25–29.9) typically live longer than people who are normal weight (BMI 18–24.9). Obesity (BMI ≤ 30.0) is associated with increased mortality from diabetes, cardiovascular disease, and certain cancers, but not other causes of death.

Flegal is associate editor of the *American Journal of Epidemiology* and a member of the Advisory Committee, Endocrinologic and Metabolic Drugs for the U.S. Food and Drug Administration; Committee on Statistics, American Heart Association; Center for Alaska Native Health Research, University of Alaska, Fairbanks; and Center for Weight and Health, University of California, Berkeley.

Jared Fogle (1977–)

Jared Fogle was born in Indianapolis. He was featured in an advertising campaign for Subway Restaurants, the national chain that specializes in selling submarine sandwiches, because of his "incredible story": When he was a junior in high school, Fogle weighed 425 pounds and wore size 6 XL shirts. He blamed the start of his weight problems on "the best birthday present of my life," a Nintendo video game system. He used a one-handed approach to playing games: one hand on the controller and one hand in a bag of chips (Nelson, 2006).

Fogle developed his own "Subway diet" by eating a 6-inch turkey sub for lunch and a 12-inch sub, potato chips, and a Diet Coke for dinner. After three months, he had lost almost 100 pounds. By the end of his diet, he had lost about 250 pounds. A former dorm-mate wrote an article about Fogle's weight-loss experience, and a reporter for *Men's Health* magazine included Fogle's Subway diet in an article entitled, "Crazy Diets That Work." He was "discovered" by the creative director at Subway's advertising agency. The restaurant chain started a regional ad campaign in 2000 featuring Fogle. The commercial carried the following disclaimer: "The Subway diet, combined with a lot of walking, worked for Jared. We're not saying this is for everyone." The campaign later went national, and Fogle has toured the country for Subway with his "fat pants." As of 2008, he has kept the weight off for 10 years.

Jeffrey M. Friedman (1954–)

Jeffrey M. Friedman was born in Orlando, Florida. He has a BS (Rensselaer Polytechnic Institute), a combined MD and PhD (Albany Medical College of Union University, 1977), and a PhD in molecular biology (The Rockefeller University, 1986). He is the Marilyn Simpson Professor and head of the Laboratory of Molecular Genetics at The Rockefeller University.

One of Friedman's publications in the journal *Science* was an essay titled "A War on Obesity, Not the Obese" and was subsequently included in *The Best American Science and Nature Writing 2004* anthology (Houghton Mifflin, 2004). Interestingly, the first paper he wrote was rejected.

Friedman's codiscovery of the hormone leptin (1994) and its role in regulating body weight have changed our understanding of the causes of human obesity. Some of his honors include election to the Institute of Medicine of the National Academies (2005), Distinguished Achievement in Metabolic Research (Bristol-Myer Myer, 2001), and the Gairdner Foundation International Award (2005).

M. R. C. Greenwood (1943–)

M. R. C. Greenwood was born in Gainesville, Florida. She has a BA from Vassar College (1968) and a PhD from The Rockefeller University (1973). She joined the faculty at the Institute of Human Nutrition at Columbia University and served in that capacity from 1969 to 1978. She returned to Vassar in 1978 and became department chair and John Guy Professor of Natural Sciences, which she held from 1986 to 1989. Greenwood moved to the University of California, Davis (UC Davis), where she was dean of Graduate Studies from 1989 to 1993; was chancellor of the University of California, Santa Cruz from 1996 to 2004; and served as provost and senior vice president of Academic Affairs for the University of California from 2004 to 2005. Greenwood is currently professor and director of the Foods for Health Program at UC Davis.

Greenwood has played a leadership role in obesity research and policy. She made significant contributions to the way science is conducted as associate director for Science at the Office of Science, Technology and Policy during the Clinton administration (1993–1995). She is one of the cofounders of The Obesity Society and a past president (1987–1988). Her honors include election to the Institute of Medicine of the National Academies (1992). She is past president (1998–1999) and board of directors member of the American Association for the Advancement of Sciences.

According to Greenwood, "The impact of the obesity and diabetes epidemic is only beginning to be felt. If we are going to significantly impact it we must enact new innovative policies in health care, urban planning and personal options. This is a massive policy opportunity and challenge. How well we do will determine the next generations' quality of life" (Greenwood, pers. comm.).

Barbara Hansen (1941–)

Barbara Hansen was born in Boston. She has a BS from the University of California, Los Angeles and a PhD from the University of Washington, Seattle. Hansen is currently professor of internal medicine and pediatrics and director of both the Center for Preclinical Research and the Center for Obesity, Diabetes, and Aging Research at the University of Tampa.

Hansen is internationally known for her research in obesity, diabetes, and aging; she has published more than 200 scientific publications. Her classic work, in the study of monkeys, demonstrated that prevention of obesity by maintaining the weight when the monkeys were young adults reduces the risk for the development of type 2 diabetes in middle and old age. Her research has added to the body of knowledge that humans (and nonhuman primates) have an extraordinary ability to regulate appetite, body weight, and body composition and that this system is influenced by age-related changes and has a strong genetic basis.

Some of her honors include membership in the Institute of Medicine of the National Academies (1981), George Bray Founder's Award (Obesity Society), and McCollum Award (American Society for Clinical Nutrition). She has served as president of The Obesity Society and of the International Association for the Study of Obesity.

According to Hansen, "The message about obesity that I like the least in today's media is—You did it to yourself,—and you can fix it! Neither is, in my view, accurate for the vast majority of overweight persons. People need extensive and multipronged new research to find ways to help mitigate the negative consequences of excessive adiposity. We must end the 'blame the patient approach' and address the underlying mechanisms of our extraordinary energy balance regulatory system" (Hansen, pers. comm.).

Marion M. Hetherington (1961–)

Marion M. Hetherington was born in Helensburgh, Scotland. She has a bachelor's degree (University of Glasgow, 1982), trained as a teacher, and received her doctorate (University of Oxford, 1987). She was awarded a Fulbright Scholarship in 1987 and worked with Dr. Barbara J. Rolls at the Johns Hopkins University School of Medicine. Her Fogarty International Fellowship allowed her to conduct research at the National Institutes of Health, which she did from 1988–1990. Hetherington currently holds the Caledonian Futures Professorship in Biopsychology at Glasgow Caledonian University, where she has served since 2005. She is president-elect for the Society for the Study of Ingestive Behavior.

Hetherington is known for her work on short-term influences on food intake, including sensory-specific satiety. Her current research focuses on early determinants of overeating in children. She has studied the impact of school-based healthy eating interventions in areas of material deprivation in Glasgow.

James O. Hill (1951–)

James O. Hill was born in Crossville, Tennessee. He has a BS from the University of Tennessee and a PhD from the University of New Hampshire. He is professor of pediatrics and medicine at the University of Colorado. Hill's research interests are studying how diet and physical activity affect body weight and how they are connected to the obesity epidemic. His work with families showed that small changes in diet and physical activity can be achieved and sustained and can help family members avoid excessive weight gain.

Hill was chair of the World Health Organization (WHO) Consultation on Obesity (1997) and president of The Obesity Society and of the American Society of Nutrition (2008), and he is a vice president of the International Association for the Study of Obesity. He established the programs Colorado on the Move (2002) and America on the Move (2003), which are regional and national health initiatives, respectively, to help tackle the obesity epidemic and inspire Americans to aim for healthier lifestyles. He believes that the small-changes approach to lifestyle modification is the best way to reverse the obesity epidemic (Hill, pers. comm.). Along with Dr. Rena Wing, he is also known for his stewardship of the National Weight Control Registry, a database of people who have lost weight.

According to Hill, "Most weight loss plans help you to lose weight but they don't help you keep it off. Weight loss and weight loss maintenance can involve different strategies and the real challenge is preventing weight regain" (Hill, pers. comm.). Hill cowrote *The Step Diet* with Dr. John C. Peters and Bonnie T. Jortberg to help people both lose weight and keep it off.

Hippocrates (460 BCE–370 BCE)

Hippocrates was born on the Greek island of Kos. He was the founder of the Hippocratic School of medicine and is known as the father of Western medicine. The Hippocratic Oath, taken by current-day physicians, refers to the ethical practice of medicine. Hippocrates was thousands of years ahead of his time when he allegedly said that taking in more food than the constitution will bear is very injurious to health when at the same time one uses no exercise to carry off this excess. He warned his fellow Greeks that sudden death is more common in those who are naturally fat than in those who are lean.

Jules Hirsch (1927–)

Jules Hirsch was born in New York City. He is one of the few physicians who went to medical school (University of Texas, Austin, 1948) without having first received a college degree. He is professor emeritus at The Rockefeller University. Some of his honors include election to the Institute of Medicine of the National Academies (1993) and a 2006 award from The Obesity Society.

Hirsch is unofficially known as "Dr. Fat Cell." His classical research found that obese people can have more fat cells, large fat cells, or a combination of the two, compared with people who are not obese. Further, he discovered that weight loss decreases the size of fat cells but not the number of these cells. He showed that different fat depots can respond differently to hormones and other compounds. Hirsch has also conducted research in psychology, reporting that people who have been obese since childhood and lose weight as adults continue to "see" themselves as fatter than they really are.

Hirsch does not "want the treatment of obesity to slip out of the scientific medical paradigm and into the realm of paramedical voodoo" (Hirsch, pers. comm.).

W. P. T. James (1938–)

W. P. T. (Phil) James was born in Liverpool, England. He has a bachelor's degree (University of London, 1959), a medical degree (UCLH, London), and a DSc (1983).

James is literally an international ambassador whose travels have highlighted the growing problem of childhood obesity in developing countries. He is founder and head of the International Obesity Taskforce (IOTF), which is part of IASO, and chair of WHO's Presidential Council of the Global Prevention Alliance. IOTF is demanding that action be taken in response to the childhood obesity crisis. James was responsible for the WHO classification of BMI for obesity. In the United States, this classification resulted in lowering the point at which adults are considered overweight from a BMI of 27 to 25.

Some of his honors include Fellow of both the Royal College of Physicians in London and in Edinburgh, Commander of the British Empire for Services to Sciences, and an honorary doctor of science from the City University of London. He was director of the Rowett Research Institute in Aberdeen, Scotland, from 1982 to 1999, which made substantial contributions to health and agricultural development around the world.

James "considers the problem of preventing obesity an enormous challenge because the fine brain control of food intake requires major environmental changes in the quality and amount of food immediately available so that the appetite drive is attempting to maintain rather than reduce weight in a free market world where huge industrial pressures incite us to do even less and eat more" (James, pers. comm.).

Robin B. Kanarek (1946–)

Robin B. Kanarek was born in Pittsburgh. She has a BA (Antioch College, 1963) and a PhD (Rutgers University, 1974). Since 1976, Kanarek has been at Tufts University and is the John Wade Professor of Psychology.

Kanarek's research focuses on the role of diet and exercise in determining behavioral consequences of neuropeptides related to food intake and on the effects of refined carbohydrates on development of obesity and diabetes. She demonstrated that in addition to leading to obesity and its related metabolic deficits, intake of high refined carbohydrates can result in impairments in cognitive behavior. Kanarek is the coauthor or editor of three books and more than 100 book chapters and papers. She is a member of the Institute of Medicine's Committee on Military Nutrition Research, associate editor of *Nutritional Neuroscience*, on the editorial boards of *Physiology and Behavior* and the *Tufts Diet and Nutrition Newsletter*, and past editor in chief of *Nutrition and Behavior*.

She believes that she is "extremely fortunate to have had the opportunity to pursue independent research in areas related to human health and to have done so with the input of outstanding students and colleagues" (Kanarek, pers. comm.).

Janet C. King (1941–)

Janet C. King was born in Red Oak, Iowa. She received a bachelor's degree from Iowa State University (1963) and a PhD from University of California, Berkeley (UC Berkeley) (1972). Upon graduation, she was immediately appointed to UC Berkeley's faculty in the Department of Nutritional Sciences and served until 1995, where she also served as chair of the department and the graduate program. King directed the U.S. Department of Agriculture (USDA) Western Human Nutrition Research Center from 1995 to 2003. She is currently a senior scientist at Children's Hospital Oakland Research Center and holds professorial appointments at UC Berkeley and UC Davis.

King is internationally known for her studies of effects of maternal nutrition and the metabolic adjustments of pregnancy. She studies effects of different diets on hormonal and metabolic pathways linked to poor pregnancy outcomes in obese women.

King has served on numerous national and international committees, including as chair of the Institute of Medicine of the National Academies Food and Nutrition Board and Committee and as a member of the Dietary Guidelines Advisory Committee. Some of her many honors include election to the Institute of Medicine National Academies (1994) and USDA Research Service Hall of Fame (2007).

When asked about her work, King said, "I have the best job in the world. I can't think of any other job where you are paid to pursue your passionate interests with talented colleagues, friends and students while potentially improving the health of mankind" (King, pers. comm.).

Ahmed Kissebah (1937–)

Ahmed Kissebah was born in Dumiat City, Egypt, also known as the "Tip of the Earth" because it is the meeting point between the Nile River and the Mediterranean Sea. He has an MD from Cairo University (1961) and a PhD from the University of London (1973). Since 1977, he has served as professor of medicine and director of the TOPS (Take Off Pounds Sensibly) Obesity and Medical Research Center at the Medical College of Wisconsin in Milwaukee.

Kissebah's most significant research contribution is his recognition that the distribution of body fat has an impact on the risk for obesity-related diseases. For example, obese women with excess fat mainly around the waist, chest, neck, and arms (upper-body obesity, or an apple shape) are at greater risk for developing type 2 diabetes than those with excess fat mainly about the thighs and buttocks (a pear shape). He used two simple measurements—circumference of the waist and the hip—to estimate body fat distribution and from these calculated the waist-to-hip ratio (WHR). In women, lower-body obesity represented a WHR of less than 0.76, and upper-body obesity represented a WHR of greater than 0.85. Kissebah's revolutionary work in this area is a benchmark for many novel ideas in obesity research. He was also part of an international team of scientists that discovered that a gene on chromosome 15 regulates inflammation, a finding that has major implications for obesity.

Kissebah is medical director of TOPS, whose members volunteer for his studies, which has allowed him to study genetics of obesity in families for more than three generations. Some of his numerous honors include Outstanding Foreign Investigator (Japan), Distinguished Armour Award (President of Egypt), Princess Margaret Distinguished Research Award (United Kingdom), and King Faisel Distinguished Scientist Award (Saudi Arabia).

When asked about his work, Kissebah responded, "I'm really grateful that I have had the opportunity to be part of the change from simple anecdotal science to in-depth, state-of-the-art technology and theorems that are bound to bring to the work a new stream of discoveries and cures that were never dreamt of" (Kissebah, pers. comm.).

C. Everett Koop (1916–)

C. Everett Koop was born in Brooklyn, New York. He has an AB from Dartmouth (1937), an MD from Cornell Medical College (1941), and a PhD from the University of Pennsylvania (1947). He is professor of surgery at Dartmouth Medical School and senior scholar of the C. Everett Koop Institute.

Koop spent the majority of his career as a pediatrician at Children's Hospital of Philadelphia, where he was the surgeon-in-chief. He is best known for starting the practice of placing warning labels on packs of cigarettes when he was surgeon general of the United States, from 1981 to 1989. He has said that, had he remained in the post of surgeon general longer, he would have tackled obesity.

He has received 35 honorary doctorates, the Legion of Honor Medal (France, 1980), the Public Health Distinguished Service Medal, and a National Academies Institute of Medicine membership (1989). Koop won an Emmy Award in 1991 for a television series on health care reform.

In 1994, Koop founded Shape Up America! (www.shapeup
.org), a nonprofit national initiative that has raised the awareness
of healthy eating and increased physical activity for obesity prevention and disease management. The organization's Web site
is an excellent resource for the public, health care professionals,
educators, and the media.

John Kral (1939–)

John Kral was born in Göteborg, Sweden. He earned both his MD
(1967) and his PhD (1976) from the University of Göteborg. His
thesis was entitled "Surgical Reduction of Adipose Tissue." Kral
was recruited to St. Lukes' Hospital Center at Columbia University in New York City, where he established the program of surgical treatment of obesity with a strong research component. He
moved to State University of New York Downstate Medical
Center in 1988 as professor of surgery and medicine and also
served as director of Surgical Services at Kings County Hospital
Center.

Kral is a pioneer in bariatric surgery and one of the cofounders in 1983 of the American Society for Bariatric Surgery. He set
high standards for bariatric surgery, including evidence-based
protocols, and is known for his visionary approach to obesity
research. Kral has said, "The study of obesity provides a foundation for understanding the entire human condition as it is
expressed in health and disease" (Kral, pers. comm.).

Ray Kroc (1902–1984)

Ray Kroc, founder of McDonald's Fast Food Restaurants, was
born in Chicago. In 1941, he was the exclusive sales agent for
milkshake mixers. These mixers could prepare six shakes at a
time. In his work, he visited Dick and Mac McDonald, owners
of a fast-food emporium in San Bernardino, California. Later,
with the brothers as partners, Kroc opened a number of McDonald's franchises. He first opened a McDonald's Restaurant in
Des Plaines, Illinois, in 1954, and eventually bought the entire
franchise in 1961 for $2.7 million. Kroc said, "You are only as
good as the people you hire" and "We take the hamburger business more seriously than anyone else." This philosophy is

exemplified by the training of new McDonald's franchise owners and managers, who participate in a 10-day training course at Hamburger University in Elk Grove, Illinois, where they receive a bachelor of Hamburgerology with a minor in french fries (*The Economist*, 2004). Kroc was the ultimate entrepreneur. "Creativity is a high falutin' word for the work I have to do between now and Tuesday."

McDonald's attracted children, in part, by using as its mascot Ronald McDonald, a clown, who was created by Willard Scott (later the NBC *Today Show* weatherman). By 1963, Ronald McDonald was recognized by 95 percent of school children—only Santa Claus was more commonly recognized (Brownell and Horgen, 2003).

McDonald's now has a global reach. The chain has sold more than 100 billion hamburgers worldwide. *The Economist* publishes the Big Mac Index using the "hamburger standard" to determine the value of the world's currencies based on the price of a Big Mac. In July 2007, the Big Mac price in the United States was $3.41; the lowest price for the Big Mac was found in Hong Kong at $1.54 and the highest was in Norway at $7.85 (*The Economist*, 2004).

Kroc also owned the San Diego Padres Major League Baseball team and he continued to be outspoken. In a 1974 game, the Padres made three errors and a costly base-running blunder. Kroc told the fans using the ballpark's public address system, "I suffer with you; I have never seen such stupid ball playing in my life" (Pace, 1984).

Shiriki Kumanyika (1945–)

Shiriki Kumanyika was born in Baltimore. She has a BA (Syracuse University, 1965), an MS (Columbia University, 1969), and a PhD (Cornell University, 1978). She is a professor in the Department of Biostatistics and Epidemiology at the University of Pennsylvania's School of Medicine.

Kumanyika has been engaged in obesity research since the mid-1980s. She founded and chairs the African American Collaborative Obesity Research Network. Her work in this capacity reflects her strong commitment to reducing obesity and related health disparities in African American communities and to increasing the engagement of African American scholars in obesity research. Kumanyika has served on numerous advisory or expert panels and work groups related to nutrition and obesity research and policy for a number of organizations, such as the National Institutes of Health, National Academies Institute of Medicine, and WHO. Some of her honors include the Population Research Prize (American Heart Association, 2005), the Symbol of H.O.P.E. (award of the *American Journal of Health*, 2006), and election to the National Academies Institute of Medicine (2003).

Kumanyika loves her work and finds it hard to be idle. She enjoys exercising and trying to keep up with the challenging global developments that affect population health and well-being.

Jack LaLanne (1914–)

Jack LaLanne was born François Henri LaLanne in San Francisco in 1914. He attended Oakland Chiropractic College in San Francisco and has come to be known as the godfather of physical fitness. In the 1930s, LaLanne invented the Smith Machine, a barbell on steel runners that could only move up and down and is used for weight training. He opened the first modern health spa in the United States in 1946 and brought exercise to television in 1951. *The Jack LaLanne Show* was broadcast on TV for 34 years; it was the longest-running TV show that was devoted to fitness. He encouraged women to lift weights even though it was thought at the time that weightlifting would make women unattractive.

LaLanne was ahead of the whole-food movement when he used to say, "If man made it, don't eat it." When asked what he thought about organic foods, LaLanne replied, "It's a bunch of bull. If you want to eat more organic that's fine, but I don't go out of my way to get to organic vegetables." When he was 70, he demonstrated his fitness by being handcuffed and shackled and swimming 1.5 miles towing 70 boats carrying 70 people from the Queen's Way Bridge in California's Long Beach Harbor to the Queen Mary. At 94 years old, he still worked out every morning for two hours. At 97 years old, Jack LaLanne was inducted into the California Hall of Fame in 2008 by California first lady Maria Shriver.

Antoine Lavoisier (1743–1794)

Antoine Lavoisier was born in Paris. During his lifetime, he studied chemistry, botany, astronomy, and mathematics at the College of Mazarin (1754–1761) and law at the University of Paris (1761–1763). He is known as the father of modern chemistry. While working for the French government, he helped develop the metric system of weights and measures. He is best known for his discovery of the role that oxygen plays in combustion. Using a calorimeter, designed by Pierre Laplace, a French physicist and mathematician, Lavoisier demonstrated that burning involves the combination of a substance with oxygen. He conducted experiments that revealed that respiration was a slow combustion of organic material using inhaled oxygen. This research formed the basis for measuring calories in food.

Unfortunately, Lavoisier used the results of others without acknowledging them. For example, Lavoisier tried to take credit for the work of Joseph Priestley, who discovered that hydrogen combined with oxygen results in water. Today, we call this plagiarism.

Lavoisier was elected into the Royal Academy of Science in 1768 but later, in 1794, he was tried as a traitor, convicted, and guillotined on May 8 by the French Revolutionists.

Lavoisier's importance to science can be summarized by the quote of one of his mathematician colleagues, M. LaGrane: "It took them only an instant to cut off his head, but France may not produce another like it in a century" (Guerlac, 1975).

Maimonides (1135–1204)

Maimonides (Moses Ben Maimon) was born in Cordoba, Spain. He was thought to be the greatest physician of his time. He treated luminaries like the Sultan Saladin and Richard the Lionheart. He wrote many medical texts, some of which have survived and have been translated into English. Comments he made about obesity still apply to the 21st century: "Obesity is harmful to the body and makes it sluggish. . . . Extremely obese individuals should travel to the seashore, do much walking in the sun, and bathe in the sea in order to lose weight. . . . Their nutrition should consist of foods that are not very nourishing such as vegetables, [especially] onions and garlic ... things which strengthen without [adding] moisture, such as roasted meat from non-fat meats. [The obese] should drink little and should perform as much [physical exercise] as possible" (Grivetti, 2003).

Jean Mayer (1920–1993)

Jean Mayer was born in Paris, the son of Andre Mayer, a famous French physiologist. He received his PhD from Yale University.

Mayer was a World War II hero. He fought with the Free French and Allied forces in North Africa, Italy, and France during World War II and was awarded 14 military decorations, including the Croix de Guerre. Mayer's scientific career was a distinguished one and spanned three continents. He was internationally known for his research in obesity and for the discovery of how hunger is regulated by the amount of glucose in the blood (i.e., glucostatic hypothesis). He was a professor at the Harvard University School of Public Health and became president and chancellor of Tufts University. He advised three U.S. presidents —Richard Nixon, Gerald Ford, and Jimmy Carter—and chaired the 1969 White House Conference on Food, Nutrition and Health. He also wrote a nutrition column for the *Boston Globe*.

Barbara J. Moore (1947–)

Barbara J. Moore was born in Paterson, New Jersey. She received her BA from Skidmore College in 1969 and then studied archeology in Israel and Greece. During that time she participated in a dig at Tell Beer Sheba, where she discovered an oven from the Iron Age. She has a PhD from Columbia University (1983), and her postdoctoral training took place at the University of California, Davis, where she worked with Dr. Judith S. Stern. From 1987 to 1989, she served as an assistant professor at Rutgers University.

Moore has extensive experience in developing programs and policy at both the private and public levels. She left academia to become general manager of Program Development for Weight Watchers International, a post she held from 1989 to 1993. She spent two years in Washington D.C., at the National

Institutes of Health and the White House Office of Science and Technology Policy. She was recruited in 1995 by former U.S. Surgeon General Dr. C. Everett Koop for his newly founded Shape Up America! initiative. In this role, she raised awareness of obesity as a health issue and has developed responsible information on weight management for the media, educators, health care professionals, and policy makers. Moore is especially concerned about the increase in childhood obesity. She believes, "Combating childhood obesity needs to become the 'moral equivalent of war' for our nation, and will require nothing less than a complete revolution in the way in which we work and live our lives, build our communities and worksites, educate and nurture ourselves and our children and set our public policy and budgetary priorities" (Moore, pers. comm.).

Jean Nidetch (1923–)

Jean Nidetch was born in Brooklyn, New York. She started the original Weight Watchers Club in the early 1960s by inviting friends to her home in Queens, New York, weekly to exchange information about how to lose weight. Through this exchange, a number of recipes were shared and developed. Some of the early recipes, such as making ketchup by boiling down tomato juice and adding the artificial sweetener Sweet'N Low or making milkshakes from powdered skim milk, ice cubes, Sweet'N Low, and flavored extracts, did not have a good taste. However, over time, the group of friends honed their recipes to improve the flavor.

According to Nidetch, "Weight Watchers does not simply give you a method of losing weight ... it is a new way of life. It is a boy whose whole life has changed because of some encouragement we gave him. This is what it is all about." She also is quoted as saying, "This is me and I am never going to change, I'll never get fat again. I don't have to suffer. I don't have to starve. I don't have to be on a diet. I am in control of myself" (Kovatch, pers. comm.). The *Ladies' Home Journal* recognized her as "one of the most important women in the United States."

Dean Ornish (1953–)

Dean Ornish was born in Dallas. He has a BA from the University of Texas at Austin and an MD from Baylor College of Medicine. He is president and founder of the Preventive Medicine Research Institute in Sausalito, California, where he holds the Safeway Chair. Over the last 30 years, Ornish directed clinical research that demonstrated that comprehensive lifestyle changes may begin to reverse even severe coronary heart disease. Medicare is now covering his weight-management program, which is based on his research.

The "Ornish program" is a lifestyle program based on eating foods low in fat, exercising, and reducing stress. Ornish recommends that only 10 percent of calories in one's diet come from fat. In contrast, the average American takes in almost 35 percent calories from fat. His work was featured in a one-hour documentary, which was broadcast on the PBS *Nova* series.

One of Ornish's more provocative statements about the negative effects of a low-carbohydrate, high-fat, high-protein diet was made when he participated in the 2002 USDA-sponsored forum called "The Diet Debate." Ornish made the following comments at this event: "Even a single meal high in fat and cholesterol makes your arteries constrict and your blood clot faster. . . . It's not just your heart that gets less blood flow . . . it can also cause sexual dysfunction. . . . What I have a hard time with is recommending that people consume meat, bacon, sausage, brie . . . when thousands of studies have shown that these increase your risk of heart disease and the most common types of cancer. . . . I'd love to be able to tell people that bacon and eggs are health foods, but they're not" (Ornish, 2000).

Ornish was appointed to the White House Commission on Complementary and Alternative Medicine Policy. In addition, he received the Kellermann Memorial Award for distinguished contributions in the field of cardiovascular disease prevention (International Academy of Cardiology). *People* magazine recognized Ornish as "one of the most interesting people of 1996." *Life* magazine recognized him as "one of the 50 most influential members of his generation."

Xavier Pi-Sunyer (1933–)

Xavier Pi-Sunyer was born in Barcelona, Spain. He has a BA (Oberlin College, 1955), an MD (Columbia College of Physicians and Surgeons, 1959) and an MPH (Harvard University School of Public Health, 1962). He is professor of Medicine at Columbia University, director of the VanItallie Center for Weight Loss and Maintenance, and chief of the Division of Endocrinology, Diabetes and Nutrition.

Pi-Sunyer's research interests are extensive and include lipid and carbohydrate metabolism, obesity, and diabetes. He has published more than 250 scientific papers and numerous review articles and book chapters.

Pi-Sunyer is known for his leadership in the field. He is past president of a number of organizations, including the American Diabetes Association, American Society for Clinical Nutrition, and Obesity Society; chairman of the Task Force on Treatment of Obesity of NIH; and a member of the board of directors for Weight Watchers Foundation. Some of his numerous honors include Fellow of the American Heart Association; Stunkard Lifetime Career Award (Obesity Society, 2000); George Bray Founders Award (Obesity Society, 2006); Luken Medal and Lecturer (American Diabetes Association, 1977); and two honorary doctorates, from the University Rome and the University of Barcelona.

Nathan Pritikin (1915–1985)

Nathan Pritikin was born in Chicago. He was a student at the University of Chicago from 1933 to 1935, but he did not receive a degree. He was diagnosed with heart disease when he was only 41. He disobeyed his doctor's advice to continue eating a diet of butter, ice cream, and steaks. Instead, he created his own diet, which was high in unrefined carbohydrates and very, very low in fat. His blood cholesterol decreased from a high of 280 to a low of 120. As a result, he no longer had heart disease. In 1976, he founded the Pritikin Longevity Center, which today offers controlled diet, counseling in lifestyle change, and exercise in a spa/resort setting.

Pritikin had an ongoing feud with Dr. Robert Atkins. The Pritikin diet was low in fat, while the Atkins diet was relatively high in fat.

Barbara J. Rolls (no date available)

Barbara J. Rolls has a BA from the University of Pennsylvania and a PhD from the University of Cambridge. She held several research fellowships at the University of Oxford, and later, in 1984, she joined the Johns Hopkins University School of Medicine faculty as a professor of psychiatry. In 1992, she became professor of nutritional sciences and currently holds the Guthrie Chair in Nutrition at the Pennsylvania State University.

She is the author of more than 200 original research articles and five books, including *The Volumetrics Weight-Control Plan: Feel Full on Fewer Calories* (HarperTorch, 2003), cowritten with Robert A. Barnett, which reached number five on the *New York Times* best-seller list in 2007, and *The Volumetrics Eating Plan* (HarperCollins, 2005), which reached the top spot on the best-seller list, also in 2007. Volumetrics is based on healthy strategies to enhance satiety. Eating soup or salad before a meal for example, will lead to eating fewer calories. This approach has been widely used in weight-loss clinics and is being incorporated into the Jenny Craig program.

Rolls is past president of both the Society for the Study of Ingestive Behavior and The Obesity Society. Some of her numerous awards include the Human Nutrition Award (American Society of Nutritional Sciences), the International Award for Modern Nutrition, honorary membership in the American Dietetic Association, and the Centrum Center for Nutrition Science Award. She is a Fellow of the American Association of the Advancement of Science.

Wim H. M. Saris (1949–)

Wim H. M. Saris was born in Zwolle, the Netherlands. He has a degree in human nutrition (1974, Wageningen University) and an MD (1979) and a PhD (1982, Catholic University of Nijmegen). He is professor and a member of the medical and health science faculty at Maastricht University. In 1992, Saris initiated the Nutrition and Toxicology Research Institute, a collaborative program focused on nutrition research, and was its first scientific director, from 1992 to 2005. He is currently a part-time corporate scientist for human nutrition for the DSM Company at the Food Ingredients site in Delft.

Saris's current obesity research is related to the experimental and public health aspects of obesity. He has written seven books and more than 350 scientific papers. He serves on national and international committees, including the Scientific Committee on Food of the European Commission and the European Technology Platform initiative Food for Life. He was president of the Netherlands Association of the Study of Obesity and the European Pediatric Exercise Society. He coordinates the European Union's (EU) sixth framework research project, DiOGenes (diet, obesity, and genes) the largest EU-funded obesity-related research program, with 33 partners.

Saris believes that the problem of obesity health is the most important global challenge, with far-reaching consequences for the society (Saris, pers. comm.).

Ethan Allen Sims (1916–)

Ethan Allen Sims was born in Newport, Rhode Island. He is the great-great-great grandson of Green Mountain Boys leader Ethan Allen. (The Green Mountain Boys were the militia of the Vermont republic in the decade prior to the American Revolution.) Sims wrote a booklet on Ethan Allen the philosopher. He has a BA from Harvard College (1938) and an MD from Columbia College of Physicians & Surgeons (1942). Sims has spent his entire academic career at the University of Vermont, starting in 1950, where he is professor of medicine emeritus. In 1991, the university named its metabolic research unit The Sims Obesity/Nutrition Research Center.

Sims is internationally known for his work in experimental obesity and diabetes. To explain the relationship between obesity and diabetes, he coined the word "diabesity." This concept describes the result of genes interacting with other genes and environmental factors to produce obesity-induced type 2 diabetes. To frame his work, he asked the question, What would happen if people who never had a weight problem deliberately got fat? His subjects, inmates at a state prison, volunteered to gain weight. Over four to six months they increased their weight by 20 to 25 percent. Some had to consume 10,000 calories a day. Two of his important conclusions were that some people put on more weight easily and take weight off with more difficulty than others. He was featured in an April 16, 2002, article in the *New York Times* entitled "Is Obesity a Disease or Just a Symptom?" Sims published many papers with his wife, Doro. To celebrate their collaborative research, they were both awarded honorary doctor of science degrees from the University of Vermont in 1990. He was also honored for his extensive contributions to clinical research by the creation of the Ethan Sims Clinical Research Feasibility Fund Award from the National Institutes of Health. The Obesity Society has honored Sims with the establishment of the Ethan Sims Young Investigator Award. His outside interests are nonmedical writing, mild exercise, music, and playing the recorder.

Sachiko St. Jeor (1941–)

Sachiko St. Jeor was born in Los Angeles. She received her PhD in nutrition from the Pennsylvania State University in 1980. She is currently professor and chief, Division of Medical Nutrition, and director of the Center for Nutrition and Metabolism in the Department of Internal Medicine at the University of Nevada School of Medicine in Reno.

St. Jeor's research has focused on metabolism. The Harris Benedict equation, developed in 1900, predicted the metabolic rate for men and women based on their age, weight, and height. With the changes in lifestyles since 1900, Dr. Mark D. Mifflin and St. Jeor developed a new equation, named after the pair, that is 5 percent more accurate and is being recommended for use today. She has developed methods for research diets used on metabolic wards and dietary intake analysis programs.

St. Jeor has been a member of many national committees, including the 1995 Dietary Guidelines Advisory Committee, Weighing the Options (National Academies, Institute of Medicine), Healthy Weight Roundtable (NIH), and Calcium Consensus Panel (American Heart Association). Some of her honors include the Medallion Award and the Award for Excellence in the Practice of Dietetic Research (American Dietetic

Association), and Fellow designations with the American Dietetic Association, American Heart Association, and Society of Behavioral Medicine.

Judith S. Stern (1943–)

Judith S. Stern was born in Brooklyn, New York. As a youth, she was active in 4-H, where she was a cherry pie–baking champion. She has a BS from Cornell University (1964) with honors and an MS and a DSc from Harvard University School of Public Health (1966, 1970, respectively), where she studied with Dr. Jean Mayer, a leading researcher in obesity.

Stern was a faculty member at The Rockefeller University from 1969 to 1974, where she worked with Dr. Jules Hirsch. She joined the faculty at UC Davis in 1975, where she is now a distinguished professor in the Departments of Nutrition and Internal Medicine.

Stern is known for her research in obesity and has published more than 270 papers in scientific journals and one popular book, *The Fast Food Diet* (Prentice-Hall, 1980). Her research has emphasized development of adipose tissue, physical activity including what happens when you suddenly stop exercising, weight control in women, and use of dietary supplements. She was president of the American Society for Clinical Nutrition and The Obesity Society. She has served on a number of national advisory committees including the Dietary Guidelines Advisory Committee and Weighing the Options (National Academies, Institute of Medicine). Stern is also known for her efforts in translating science for the public. She was a contributing editor and columnist for *Vogue* magazine and has written more than 150 popular articles.

Stern's honors include the New York State 4-H Community Service State award (1960); election to the National Academies Institute of Medicine (1995); fellow of the American Association for the Advancement of Science (2009); and, along with Dr. Richard L. Atkinson, being the first corecipient of the Atkinson-Stern Award for Distinguished Public Service (The Obesity Society, 2006). Stern states, "Obesity is the #1 threat to our health in the USA. Yet, our federal government discriminates against obesity and people with obesity. It spends more than twice the amount of money for research in heart disease and CVD [cardio-vascular disease]."

Albert J. Stunkard (1922–)

Albert J. (Mickey) Stunkard obtained his MD from Columbia University in 1945. He is professor of psychiatry emeritus at the University of Pennsylvania School of Medicine.

Stunkard is a pioneer in the study of eating behavior. He was first to describe "binge eating" and develop a treatment for it (Stunkard and Allison, 2002).

Stunkard was also the first researcher to describe "night-eating syndrome" (NES), a new eating disorder linked to obesity. NES is associated with not being hungry in the morning but being hungry in the evening and experiencing insomnia whereby one wakes up frequently during the night to eat.

Stunkard is currently conducting a large-scale study of the growth and development of children at high risk of obesity. The children in the study have been participating since three months of age. The children's mothers are either lean or obese. Some of his major findings are related to food intake and body weight during the first year of life, the importance of sucking behavior at three months in predicting body weight and adiposity five years later, and the importance of rate of food intake in determining adiposity in subjects at high risk of obesity.

Two of Stunkard's many honors include election to the National Academies Institute of Medicine member (1988) and creation of the Stunkard Lifetime Achievement Award (Obesity Society, 2003) to recognize individuals who have made outstanding contributions to the field of obesity.

Stunkard was quoted as saying, "I began my career in obesity research at the beginning of the obesity epidemic and have continued it aggressively as the epidemic expanded. Perhaps when I stop working on obesity waistlines will return to normal" (Stunkard, pers. comm.).

Oprah Winfrey (1954–)

Oprah Winfrey was born in Kosciusko, Mississippi, into abject poverty. She studied speech and the performing arts at

Tennessee State University. She got a job in radio while in high school and coanchored the local evening news when she was 19—the first black woman to hold that job.

She is the multiple–Emmy award winning host of the *Oprah Winfrey Show*, the highest-rated talk show in TV history. Winfrey has been called the "ultimate media icon." CNN has declared her the "world's most powerful woman." *Vanity Fair* magazine wrote that she has had "more influence on the culture than any university president, politician, or religious leader, except perhaps the Pope" (Harrow, 2004). Winfrey continues to fight "the battle of the bulge." She has gone public with how difficult it is to lose weight, even considering that Winfrey is one of the wealthiest people in the United States. She has a personal trainer (Bob Greene) and a chef. She has said that if there was a pill or a diet that magically caused weight loss, she would take it (Winfrey, 1997).

Winfrey is committed to making the world a better place. In 1998, she started the Oprah's Angel Network. This charity encourages people to make a difference in the lives of the underprivileged around the world. She also established the Oprah Winfrey Leadership Academy for Girls in Johannesburg, South Africa.

Rena Wing (1945–)

Rena Wing was born in New York. She has a BA from Connecticut College (1967) and a master's and doctorate from Harvard University (1971). Wing spent almost 25 years at the University of Pittsburgh before moving to Brown University's Alpert Medical School in 1998. Currently, she is professor of psychiatry and human behavior and director of the Weight Control and Diabetes Research Center at Miriam Hospital.

Wing is internationally known for her research on behavioral treatment of obesity and its application to type 2 diabetes. She was responsible for designing and overseeing the lifestyle intervention that was used in the NIH-funded Diabetes Prevention Program, which was effective in reducing the risk of developing diabetes. In 1994, Wing developed the National Weight Control Registry (NWCR) with Dr. James Hill. The NWCR includes more than 5,000 individuals who have been successful in losing weight and maintaining it and has been very important in increasing understanding of long-term weight-loss maintenance.

Wing is known for her leadership in obesity and diabetes. She was a member of the NIH Task Force on Prevention and Treatment of Obesity; a member of the Council of the National Institute of Diabetes, Digestive and Kidney Diseases at NIH; and president of the Society of Behavioral Medicine. She has published more than 250 peer-reviewed articles in the area of obesity treatment and prevention. Her honors include the TOPS Award for outstanding achievement (Obesity Society, 2001) and the Distinguished Contributions award (Behavioral Medicine and Psychology Council of the American Diabetes Association).

Wing believes, "We have made progress in proving that even modest weight loss has tremendous health benefits and helping people achieve initial weight losses; now we need to focus on improving weight loss maintenance" (Wing, pers. comm.).

References

Allison, David. Interview with author, 2008.

"Big Mac's Makeover." *The Economist*, Business Section, October 14, 2004.

Blackburn, George. Interview with author, 2008.

Blair, Steven N. Interview with author, 2008.

Bouchard Claude. Interview with author, 2008

Brody, Jane. "No Gimmicks: Eat Less and Exercise More." *New York Times*, January 1, 2008.

Brody, Jane. American Entertainment International Speakers Bureau. www.aeispeakers.com.

Brownell, K. D., and K. B. Horgen. *Food Fight: The Inside Story of The Food Industry, America's Obesity Crisis, and What We Can Do about It.* New York: McGraw-Hill, 2003.

Campos, Paul. *The Obesity Myth.* New York: Gotham Books, 2004, 192–193.

Clinton, William Jefferson. Interview with Dr. Sanjay Gupta, CNN, August 7, 2005.

Drewnowski, Adam. Interview with author, 2008.

Dwyer, Johanna. Interview with author, 2008.

Flegal, Katherine. Interview with author, 2008.

"The Global Epidemic of Obesity: An Interview with William Dietz." eJournal USA: Global Issues, January 2005, 16–19.

Greenwood, M. R. C. Interview with author, 2008.

Grivetti, Louis J. Spring Seminar Series, Oxford Brookes University, 2003.

Guerlac, Henry. *Antoine-Laurent Lavoiser: Chemist and Revolutionary.* New York: Scribner, 1975.

Hansen, Barbara. Interview with author, 2008.

Harrow, Susan. *The Ultimate Guide to Getting Booked on Oprah.* Larkspur, CA: Harrow Communications, 2004.

Hill, James O. Interview with author, 2008.

Hirsch, Jules. Interview with author, 2008.

James, W. P. T. Interview with author, 2008.

Kanarek, Robin. Interview with author, 2008.

King, Janet. Interview with author, 2008.

Kissebah, Ahmed. Interview with author, 2008.

Kovatch, Karen. Weight Watchers International. Interview with author, 2008.

Kral, John. Interview with author, 2008.

Leith, William. "Robert Atkins. Diet Guru Who Grew Fat on the Proceeds of the Carbohydrate Revolution." *The Guardian*, April 19, 2003.

Moore, Barbara J. Interview with author, 2008.

Nelson, A. "Jared Chews the Fat at MU." *Columbia Daily Tribune*, January 18, 2006.

Ornish, Dean. "The Great Diet Debate—What Is the Best Way to Stay Slim." United States Department of Agriculture, February 24, 2000.

Pace, Eric. "Ray A. Kroc Dies at 81; Builds McDonald's Chain. *New York Times* Obituary, January 15, 1984.

Saris, Wim. H. M. Interview with author, 2008.

Stunkard, A. J., and K. C. Allison. "Two Forms of Disordered Eating in Obesity: Binge Eating and Night Eating." *International Journal of Obesity* 27 (2002):1–12.

Stunkard, A. J. Interview with author, 2008.

Winfrey, Oprah. *Oprah: Make the Connection*, Video, Director: Holly Dale, 1997.

Wing, Rena. Interview with author, 2008.

6

Data and Documents

L isted here are selected facts and figures and tools for assessing and managing obesity that were current as of 2009. More detailed information about each of these items is provided in chapters 1 through 3.

Data

- An estimated 65 percent of adult Americans are overweight, and 30 percent—or 72 million—are obese (Ogden et al. 2007). Figure 6.1 shows increasing percentage of obesity by state in the United States from 1990 to 2006. The dramatic increase in obesity in the United States is illustrated by maps that show the rise in prevalence of obesity across each state from 1990 to 2006.
- Overweight and obesity increases risk for developing more than 35 major diseases, heart disease, hypertension, type 2 diabetes, respiratory problems, osteoarthritis, gallbladder disease, and certain types of cancer (NHLBI 1998).
- The most immediate consequence of overweight as perceived by children is social discrimination. This experience is associated with poor self-esteem and depression (HHS 2001).
- Attempting to lose weight is a common pursuit for many Americans. A study published in 2005 reported that 46 percent of U.S. women and 33 percent of U.S. men said they were trying to lose weight (Bish et al. 2005).

FIGURE 6.1
Obesity Trends* Among U.S. Adults
Behavioral Risk Factor Surveillance System (BRFSS), 1990, 1998, 2007
(*BMI ≥ 30, or about 30 lbs. overweight for 5′4″ person)

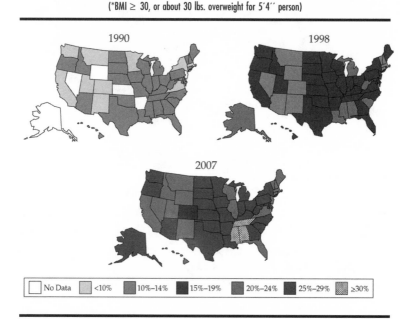

| No Data | <10% | 10%–14% | 15%–19% | 20%–24% | 25%–29% | ≥30% |

Source: Centers for Disease Control and Prevention. [Online information, retrieved 01/29/09] http://www.cdc.gov/nccdphp/dnpa/obesity/trend/maps/index.htm

- The success rate for dieting is approximately 3 to 5 percent (NHLBI 1998).
- At this time no reliable data are available to show that any diet plan will work better than the others over the long term (Bessesen 2008).
- One pound of body fat stores about 3,500 calories.
- A 15-minute brisk walk uses 100 kilocalories (Kcal) of energy.
- A Burger King Double Whopper with Cheese and a Jack in the Box Bacon Ultimate Cheeseburger each contain about 1,000 calories (Burger King 2008; Jack in the Box 2008).
- Americans eat more food than ever before—an average increase of more than 300 calories per day compared with that consumed in 1985 (Putnam, Allshouse, and Kantor 2002).

- In the 1950s, the standard-size Coca Cola was about 6 ounces. At many U.S. convenience stores today, 64-ounce soft drinks (or 2 quarts) are common.
- In 2000, a historical moment occurred when the estimate of the number of overweight people in the world exceeded the number of people suffering from malnutrition (Gardner and Halweil 2000).
- One of the most alarming trends in recent years has been the rise in worldwide childhood obesity. At least 20 million children under the age of five years are overweight (WHO 2008).
- Type 2 diabetes, closely linked to overweight and obesity and previously considered an adult disease, has increased dramatically in children and adolescents (CDC 2007).
- In 1942, the Metropolitan Life Insurance Company's standard height-weight tables for men and women, shown in Table 6.1, were transformed from a record of national averages of weight in relation to age, sex, and height to become widely used for determining "ideal" body weights.
- Body mass index (BMI) equals a person's weight in kilograms divided by height in meters squared (BMI = kg/m^2). Table 6.2 provides precalculated values. One uses the table finding his or her height in the left-hand column and move across the row to his or her weight. The number at the top of that intersecting column is the BMI for that person's height and weight.
- Overweight is defined as a BMI of equal to or greater than 25. Obesity is defined as a BMI of 30 and above. A BMI of 30 is about 30 pounds overweight.
- Skinfold tests estimate body composition from caliper measurements of a fold of skin, which are then used in the Siri equation to estimate percentage of fat. In women, the triceps, suprailiac, and thigh skinfolds are measured, and in men, the chest, abdominal, and thigh skinfolds are used. The Jackson and Pollock (1978) equation for men and the Jackson, Pollock, and Ward (1980) equation for women have been extensively cross-validated with other body composition measures (see Table 6.3). Standard errors range from 3.6 percent to 3.8 percent. The potential

TABLE 6.1
1942–1943 Metropolitan Life's Height and Weight Tables

Table 6.1a **Proposed range of ideal weights for women, ages 25 and over, Metropolitan Life Insurance Company**

Height (with shoes)	Weight in pounds (as ordinarily dressed)		
	Small frame	Medium frame	Large frame
5'0"	105–13	112–20	119–29
5'1"	107–15	114–22	121–31
5'2"	110–18	117–25	124–35
5'3"	113–21	120–28	127–38
5'4"	116–25	124–32	131–42
5'5"	119–28	127–35	133–45
5'6"	123–32	130–40	138–50
5'7"	126–36	134–44	142–54
5'8"	129–39	137–47	145–58
5'9"	133–43	141–51	149–62
5'10"	136–47	145–55	152–66
5'11"	139–50	148–58	155–69
6'0"	141–53	151–63	160–74

Table 6.1b **Ideal weights for men, ages 25 and over, Metropolitan Life Insurance Company**

Height (with shoes)	Weight in pounds (as ordinarily dressed)		
	Small frame	Medium frame	Large frame
5'2"	116–25	124–33	131–42
5'3"	119–28	127–36	133–44
5'4"	122–32	130–40	137–49
5'5"	126–36	134–44	141–53
5'6"	129–39	137–47	145–57
5'7"	133–43	141–51	149–62
5'8"	136–47	145–56	153–66
5'9"	140–51	149–60	157–70
5'10"	144–55	153–64	161–75
5'11"	148–59	157–68	165–80
6'0"	152–64	161–73	169–85
6'1"	157–69	166–78	174–90
6'2"	163–75	171–84	179–96
6'3"	168–80	176–89	184–202

Source: Metropolitan Life Insurance Company. "Ideal Weights for Men 1942." *Statistical Bulletin of the Metropolitan Life Insurance Company* 23 (1942): 6–8. Metropolitan Life Insurance Company. "Ideal Weights for Women 1943." *Statistical Bulletin of the Metropolitan Life Insurance Company* 24 (1943): 6–8. Table graphics downloaded from Czerniawski.

TABLE 6.2
Body Mass Index Table

	Normal						Overweight					Obese										Extreme Obesity														
BMI	19	20	21	22	23	24	25	26	27	28	29	30	31	32	33	34	35	36	37	38	39	40	41	42	43	44	45	46	47	48	49	50	51	52	53	54
Height (inches)												Body Weight (pounds)																								
58	91	96	100	105	110	115	119	124	129	134	138	143	148	153	158	162	167	172	177	181	186	191	196	201	205	210	215	220	224	229	234	239	244	248	253	258
59	94	99	104	109	114	119	124	128	133	138	143	148	153	158	163	168	173	178	183	188	193	198	203	208	212	217	222	227	232	237	242	247	252	257	262	267
60	97	102	107	112	118	123	128	133	138	143	148	153	158	163	168	174	179	184	189	194	199	204	208	215	220	225	230	235	240	245	250	255	261	266	271	276
61	100	106	111	116	122	127	132	137	143	148	153	158	164	169	175	180	186	191	196	202	207	211	217	222	227	232	238	243	248	254	259	264	269	275	280	285
62	104	109	115	120	126	131	136	142	147	153	158	164	169	175	180	186	191	196	202	207	213	218	224	229	235	240	246	251	256	262	267	273	278	284	289	295
63	107	113	118	124	130	135	141	146	152	158	163	169	175	180	186	191	197	203	208	214	220	225	231	237	242	248	254	259	265	270	278	282	287	293	299	304
64	110	116	122	128	134	140	145	151	157	163	169	174	180	186	192	197	204	209	215	221	227	232	238	244	250	256	262	267	273	279	285	291	296	302	308	314
65	114	120	126	132	138	144	150	156	162	168	174	180	186	192	198	204	210	216	222	228	234	240	246	252	258	264	270	276	282	288	294	300	306	312	318	324
66	118	124	130	136	142	148	155	161	167	173	179	186	192	198	204	210	216	223	229	235	241	247	253	260	266	272	278	284	291	297	303	309	315	322	328	334
67	121	127	134	140	146	153	159	166	172	178	185	191	198	204	211	217	223	230	236	242	249	255	261	268	274	280	287	293	299	306	312	319	325	331	338	344
68	125	131	138	144	151	158	164	171	177	184	190	197	203	210	216	223	230	236	243	249	256	262	269	276	282	289	295	302	308	315	322	328	335	341	348	354
69	128	135	142	149	155	162	169	176	182	189	196	203	209	216	223	230	236	243	250	257	263	270	277	284	291	297	304	311	318	324	331	338	345	351	358	365
70	132	139	146	153	160	167	174	181	188	195	202	209	216	222	229	236	243	250	257	264	271	278	285	292	299	306	313	320	327	334	341	348	355	362	369	376
71	136	143	150	157	165	172	179	186	193	200	208	215	222	229	236	243	250	257	265	272	279	286	293	301	308	315	322	329	338	343	351	358	365	372	379	386
72	140	147	154	162	169	177	184	191	199	206	213	221	228	235	242	250	258	265	272	279	287	294	302	309	316	324	331	338	346	353	361	368	375	383	390	397
73	144	151	159	166	174	182	189	197	204	212	219	227	235	242	250	257	265	272	280	288	295	302	310	318	325	333	340	348	355	363	371	378	386	393	401	408
74	148	155	163	171	179	186	194	202	210	218	225	233	241	249	256	264	272	280	287	295	303	311	319	326	334	342	350	358	365	373	381	389	396	404	412	420
75	152	160	168	176	184	192	200	208	216	224	232	240	248	256	264	272	279	287	295	303	311	319	327	335	343	351	359	367	375	383	391	399	407	415	423	431
76	156	164	172	180	189	197	205	213	221	230	238	246	254	263	271	279	287	295	304	312	320	328	336	344	353	361	369	377	385	394	402	410	418	426	435	443

Source: National Heart, Lung and Blood Institute. "Clinical Guidelines on the Identification, Evaluation, and Treatment of Overweight and Obesity in Adults—the Evidence Report." 1998. [Online information; retrieved 1/12/09.] http://www.nhlbi.nih.gov/guidelines/obesity/bmi_tbl.pdf.

TABLE 6.3
Determining Percentage of Body Fat Using Skinfold Calipers

Females:	Body density = 1.0994921 − 0.0009929 * sum + 0.0000023 * sum^2 − 0.0001392 * age
(sum means the sum of triceps, suprailiac, and thigh skinfold measurements)	
Males:	Body density = 1.1093800 − 0.0008267 * sum + 0.0000016 * sum^2 − 0.0002574 * age
(sum means the sum of chest, abdominal, and thigh skinfold measures; *=times (multiplied by)	

How to measure body area skinfolds:

Chest—A diagonal pinch halfway between the armpit and the nipple
Suprailiac—A diagonal pinch just above the front forward protrusion of the hip bone
Abdominal—A vertical pinch about one inch from the belly button
Thigh—A vertical pinch halfway between the knee and top of the thigh
Triceps—A vertical pinch halfway between the shoulder and the elbow

Estimation of percentage of fat with the Siri equation

A commonly used equation for estimating percentage of fat from body density is the 1961 Siri formula (below). Body density can be determined with skinfold measurement as follows:
Siri percentage fat = [(495/body density) − 450] * 100
A limitation to this formula is that it assumes the density of fat-free mass to remain a constant across the population. Actual percentage of fat tends to be slightly higher than the measured percentage in lean, muscular individuals and lower in obese individuals.

Sources: Jackson and Pollock (1978), "Generalized Equations for Predicting Body Density of Men." *Br J Nutr* 40(3): 497–504.
Jackson, Pollock, and Ward (1980), "Generalized Equations for Predicting Body Density of Women." *Med Sci Sports Exerc* 12(3): 175–181.
Siri (1993). "Body Composition from Fluid Spaces and Density: Analysis of Methods. 1961." *Nutrition* 9(5): 480–491; discussion 480, 492.

errors are increased when these equations are used on populations who are young or old, very lean and muscular, or obese.

- "MyPyramid Calorie Levels" is a chart that shows the appropriate calories needed for males and females by age and activity level (see Table 6.4).
- "MyPyramid Food Intake Patterns" identifies suggested amounts of food to consume from the various food groups at 12 different calorie levels (see Table 6.5).
- A daily food record helps people keep track of when they eat, what and how much they are eating, and their hunger level (see Table 6.6).

TABLE 6.4
MyPyramid Calorie Levels

Activity level	MALES			Activity level	FEMALES		
	Sedentary*	Mod. active*	Active*		Sedentary*	Mod. active*	Active*
AGE				AGE			
2	1000	1000	1000	2	1000	1000	1000
3	1000	1400	1400	3	1000	1200	1400
4	1200	1400	1600	4	1200	1400	1400
5	1200	1400	1600	5	1200	1400	1600
6	1400	1600	1800	6	1200	1400	1600
7	1400	1600	1800	7	1200	1600	1800
8	1400	1600	2000	8	1400	1600	1800
9	1600	1800	2000	9	1400	1600	1800
10	1600	1800	2200	10	1400	1800	2000
11	1800	2000	2200	11	1600	1800	2000
12	1800	2200	2400	12	1600	2000	2200
13	2000	2200	2600	13	1600	2000	2200
14	2000	2400	2800	14	1800	2000	2400
15	2200	2600	3000	15	1800	2000	2400
16	2400	2800	3200	16	1800	2000	2400
17	2400	2800	3200	17	1800	2000	2400
18	2400	2800	3200	18	1800	2000	2400
19–20	2600	2800	3000	19–20	2000	2200	2400
21–25	2400	2800	3000	21–25	2000	2200	2400
26–30	2400	2600	3000	26–30	1800	2000	2400
31–35	2400	2600	3000	31–35	1800	2000	2200
36–40	2400	2600	2800	36–40	1800	2000	2200
41–45	2200	2600	2800	41–45	1800	2000	2200
46–50	2200	2400	2800	46–50	1800	2000	2200
51–55	2200	2400	2800	51–55	1600	1800	2200
56–60	2200	2400	2600	56–60	1600	1800	2200
61–65	2000	2400	2600	61–65	1600	1800	2000
66–70	2000	2200	2600	66–70	1600	1800	2000
71–75	2000	2200	2600	71–75	1600	1800	2000
76 and up	2000	2200	2400	76 and up	1600	1800	2000

*Calorie levels are based on the Estimated Energy Requirements (EER) and activity levels from the Institute of Medicine Dietary Reference Intakes Macronutrients Report, 2002.

SEDENTARY = less than 30 minutes a day of moderate physical activity in addition to daily activities.

MOD. ACTIVE = at least 30 minutes up to 60 minutes a day of moderate physical activity in addition to daily activities.

ACTIVE = 60 or more minutes a day of moderate physical activity in addition to daily activities.

Source: USDA (2005).

TABLE 6.5
MyPyramid Food Intake Patterns

MyPyramid

Food Intake Patterns

The suggested amounts of food to consume from the basic food groups, subgroups, and oils to meet recommended nutrient intakes at 12 different calorie levels. Nutrient and energy contributions from each group are calculated according to the nutrient-dense forms of foods in each group (e.g., lean meats and fat-free milk). The table also shows the discretionary calorie allowance that can be accommodated within each calorie level, in addition to the suggested amounts of nutrient-dense forms of foods in each group.

Daily Amount of Food From Each Group

Calorie Level[1]	1,000	1,200	1,400	1,600	1,800	2,000	2,200	2,400	2,600	2,800	3,000	3,200
Fruits[2]	1 cup	1 cup	1.5 cups	1.5 cups	1.5 cups	2 cups	2 cups	2 cups	2 cups	2.5 cups	2.5 cups	2.5 cups
Vegetables[3]	1 cup	1.5 cups	1.5 cups	2 cups	2.5 cups	2.5 cups	3 cups	3 cups	3.5 cups	3.5 cups	4 cups	4 cups
Grains[4]	3 oz-eq	4 oz-eq	5 oz-eq	5 oz-eq	6 oz-eq	6 oz-eq	7 oz-eq	8 oz-eq	9 oz-eq	10 oz-eq	10 oz-eq	10 oz-eq
Meat and Beans[5]	2 oz-eq	3 oz-eq	4 oz-eq	5 oz-eq	5 oz-eq	5.5 oz-eq	6 oz-eq	6.5 oz-eq	6.5 oz-eq	7 oz-eq	7 oz-eq	7 oz-eq
Milk[6]	2 cups	2 cups	2 cups	3 cups	3 cups	3 cups	3 cups	3 cups	3 cups	3 cups	3 cups	3 cups
Oils[7]	3 tsp	4 tsp	4 tsp	5 tsp	5 tsp	6 tsp	6 tsp	7 tsp	8 tsp	8 tsp	10 tsp	11 tsp
Discretionary calorie allowance[8]	165	171	171	132	195	267	290	362	410	426	512	648

[1] Calorie Levels are set across a wide range to accommodate the needs of different individuals. The attached table "Estimated Daily Calorie Needs" can be used to help assign individuals to the food intake pattern at a particular calorie level.

[2] Fruit Group includes all fresh, frozen, canned, and dried fruits and fruit juices. In general, 1 cup of fruit or 100% fruit juice, or 1/2 cup of dried fruit can be considered as 1 cup from the fruit group.

[3] Vegetable Group includes all fresh, frozen, canned, and dried vegetables and vegetable juices. In general, 1 cup of raw or cooked vegetables or vegetable juice, or 2 cups of raw leafy greens can be considered as 1 cup from the vegetable group.

[4] Grains Group includes all foods made from wheat, rice, oats, cornmeal, barley, such as bread, pasta, oatmeal, breakfast cereals, tortillas, and grits. In general, 1 slice of bread, 1 cup of ready-to-eat cereal, or 1/2 cup of cooked rice, pasta, or cooked cereal can be considered as 1 ounce equivalent from the grains group. **At least half of all grains consumed should be whole grains.**

[5] Meat & Beans Group in general, 1 ounce of lean meat, poultry, or fish, 1 egg, 1 Tbsp. peanut butter, 1/4 cup cooked dry beans, or 1/2 ounce of nuts or seeds can be considered as 1 ounce equivalent from the meat and beans group.

[6] Milk Group includes all fluid milk products and foods made from milk that retain their calcium content, such as yogurt and cheese. Foods made from milk that have little to no calcium, such as cream cheese, cream, and butter, are not part of the group. Most milk group choices should be fat-free or low-fat. In general, 1 cup of milk or yogurt, 1 1/2 ounces of natural cheese, or 2 ounces of processed cheese can be considered as 1 cup from the milk group.

[7] Oils include fats from many different plants and from fish that are liquid at room temperature, such as canola, corn, olive, soybean, and sunflower oil. Some foods are naturally high in oils, like nuts, olives, some fish, and avocados. Foods that are mainly oil include mayonnaise, certain salad dressings, and soft margarine.

[8] Discretionary Calorie Allowance is the remaining amount of calories in a food intake pattern after accounting for the calories needed for all food groups—using forms of foods that are fat-free or low-fat and with no added sugars.

Source: USDA (2005).

TABLE 6.6
Example of a Daily Food Record

Time	Amount	Food Eaten	How Prepared	How Hungry Am I? (0 = not hungry, 5 = very hungry)
6 a.m.	1 cup	1% milk	In bowl	1
	2 cups	Cheerios	In bowl	
	2 tbsp	White sugar	In bowl	
	2 cup	Black coffee	Brewed	
	2 tbsp	fat-free nondairy creamer	In coffee	
10 a.m.	2–3 inch diameter	Chocolate chip cookies	From grocery bakery	3
Noon	2 slices	Ham, deli sliced	In sandwich	4
	1 slice	American cheese	In sandwich	
	1 leaf, 2 slices	Iceberg lettuce, pickle slices	In sandwich	
	1 tsp	Mustard	In sandwich	
	2 tbsp	Kraft real mayonnaise	In sandwich	
	2 slices	Orowheat 100% whole-wheat bread	In sandwich	
	1 bag (1.4 oz.)	Doritos Corn Chips		
	16 oz.	Sprite	Bottle	
5 p.m.	2 cups	Lasagna noodles with meat Stouffer's frozen dinner	Baked	4
	2 slices	White Italian bread	Toasted	
	2 tsp	Promise light margarine	Spread on toast	
8 p.m.	2 cups	Ben and Jerry's Vanilla ice cream	In bowl	2

TABLE 6.7
Types of Diet Plans, with Claims and Advantages

Diet Plan Characteristics	Examples	Claims/Advantages
Calorie controlled, low fat, high carbohydrates	Weight Watchers, volumetrics, Ornish, Pritikin	Balanced plan Ease into maintenance
High protein, high fat, low carbohydrates	Atkins, Scarsdale, Carb Addicts, Sugar Busters Quick Weight Loss, Protein Power, South Beach—initial stage	Quick initial weight loss No measuring No hunger
High protein, moderate fat, moderate carbohydrates	Zone, South Beach—later stages	Use fat for energy No hunger Include a wide variety of foods
Meal replacement	Jenny Craig, Nutrisystems	Portion controlled No meal preparation
Liquid protein shakes/bars	Optifast, Medifast, Health Maintenance Resources, Cambridge, Slim-Fast	Minimal dealing with food Quick initial weight loss
Others: May have very specific recommendations that make them unique; however, diet composition is generally similar to low fat or low carbohydrate, low calorie	Fit for Life, Food Combining, Fat Flush, Eat for Your Blood Type, Suzanne Somers	Quick initial weight loss Structured plan

- The chart shown in Table 6.7 helps sort through the various types of diets that exist today. It lists some of the most common diet plans, examines their advantages and disadvantages, and provides the dietary basis behind their potential benefits.
- The National Heart, Lung and Blood Institute (NHLBI) Expert Panel's treatment decision process provides a step-by-step approach to managing overweight and obese patients with its algorithm for the assessment and treatment of overweight and obesity (see Figure 6.2).
- *The Practical Guide to the Identification, Evaluation, and Treatment of Overweight and Obesity in Adults* (NHLBI and NAASO 2000) is based on the results from scientific studies. Figure 6.3 shows how evidence-based methodology ranks scientific evidence according to freedom from bias.

FIGURE 6.2
Algorithm for the Assessment and Treatment of Obesity

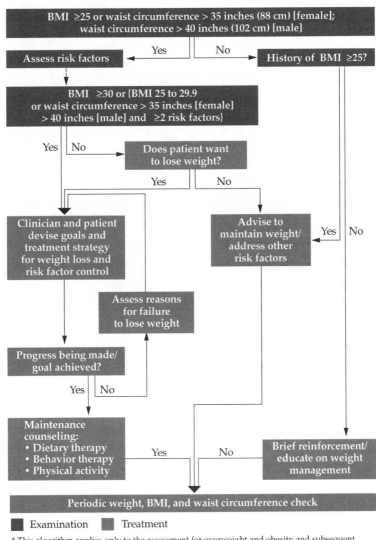

Examination ▪ Treatment

* This algorithm applies only to the assessment for overweight and obesity and subsequent decisions based on that assessment. It does not reflect any initial overall assessment for other cardiovascular risk factors that are indicated.

Source: NHLBI and North American Association for the Study of Obesity (2000).

FIGURE 6.3
Evidence Categories

Evidence Category	Source of Evidence	Definition
A	Randomized controlled trials (rich body of data)	Evidence is from endpoints of well-designed RCTs (or trials that depart only minimally from randomization) that provide a consistent pattern of findings in the population for which the recommendation is made. Category A therefore requires substantial numbers of studies involving substantial numbers of participants.
B	Randomized controlled trials (limited body of data)	Evidence is from endpoints of intervention studies that include only a limited number of RCTs, post hoc or subgroup analysis of RCTs, or meta-analysis of RCTs. In general, Category B pertains when few randomized trials exist, they are small in size, and the trial results are somewhat inconsisten, or the trials were undertaken in a population that differs from the target population of the recommendation.
C	Nonrandomized trials Observational Studies	Evidence is from outcomes of uncontrolled or nonrandomized trials or from observational studies.
D	Panel Consensus Judgment	Expert judgment is based on the panel's synthesis of evidence from experimental research described in the literature and/or derived from the consensus of panel members based on clinical derived from the consensus of panel members based on clinical criteria. The category is used only in cases where the provision of some guidance was deemed valuable but an adequately compelling clinical literature addressing the subject of the recommendation was deemed insufficient to justify placement in one of the other categories (A through C).

Source: from *The Practical Guide to the Identification, Evaluation, and Treatment of Overweight and Obesity in Adults.* National Heart, Lung, and Blood Institute and North American Association for the Study of Obesity. Bethesda, MD: National Institutes of Health; 2000. NIH Publication number 00–4084, October 2000.

Documents

Clinical Guidelines on the Identification, Evaluation, and Treatment of Overweight and Obesity in Adults: The Evidence Report

At the time these guidelines were released in September 1998 by NHLBI, they were a state-of-the-art review of the scientific evidence on the effects of treatment of overweight and obesity. The guidelines prescribed a new approach for the assessment of overweight and obesity. According to the report, assessment of overweight required evaluation of three measures—BMI, waist circumference, and an individual's risk factors for health conditions associated with obesity. The guidelines also formally established the risks associated with excess weight. The message that the guidelines were meant to convey to physicians and the public was that overweight and obesity should be taken seriously as a medical condition.

In order to recommend the most appropriate treatment, the NHLBI Expert Panel conducted an extensive review of the scientific evidence on overweight and obesity. Evidence from nearly 400 randomized controlled trials (RCTs) was considered. Their recommendations used an evidence-based methodology whereby evidence is ranked according to freedom from bias. Figure 6.3 summarizes the categories of evidence and includes a definition for each category.

The primary purpose of the report was to provide standards for physicians and health professionals, health care policy makers, and researchers to use for assessing and treating overweight and obese patients.

Individuals can access the full report, the evidence tables, a BMI calculator and BMI table, and additional practical information from the NHLBI Web site at http://www.nhlbi.nih.gov/guidelines/obesity/index.htm.

Print copies are available by writing to the NHLBI Information Center

P.O. Box 30105

Bethesda, MD 20824-0105.

NHLBI is in the process of developing new evidence-based updates of the existing guidelines for high blood pressure, cholesterol, and obesity as elements of integrated, comprehensive guidelines for reducing cardiovascular disease. The expected release date for an update of the current obesity guidelines is Spring 2010.

The abbreviated table of contents below shows the extent of the entire report. The excerpt "Summary of Evidence-Based Recommendations" is taken from the Executive Summary section beginning on page xi.

Table of Contents

Executive Summary
A. Advantages of Weight Loss

The recommendation to treat overweight and obesity is based not only on evidence that relates obesity to increased mortality but also on RCT evidence that weight loss reduces risk factors for disease. Thus, weight loss may not only help control diseases worsened by obesity, it may also help decrease the likelihood of developing these diseases. The panel reviewed RCT evidence to determine the effect of weight loss on blood pressure and hypertension, serum/plasma lipid concentrations, and fasting blood glucose and fasting insulin. Recommendations focusing on these conditions underscore the advantages of weight loss.

1. Blood Pressure

To evaluate the effect of weight loss on blood pressure and hypertension, 76 articles reporting RCTs were considered for inclusion in these guidelines. Of the 45 accepted articles, 35 were lifestyle trials and 10 were pharmacotherapy trials. There is strong and consistent evidence from these lifestyle trials in both overweight hypertensive and nonhypertensive patients that weight loss produced by lifestyle modifications reduces blood pressure levels. Limited evidence exists that decreases in abdominal fat will reduce blood pressure in overweight nonhypertensive individuals, although not independent of weight loss, and there is considerable evidence that increased aerobic activity to increase cardio-respiratory fitness reduces blood pressure (independent of weight loss). There is also suggestive evidence from randomized trials that weight loss produced by most weight loss medications, except for sibutramine, in combination with adjuvant lifestyle modifications will be accompanied by reductions in blood pressure. Based on a review of the evidence from the 45 RCT blood pressure articles, the panel makes the following recommendation:

Weight loss is recommended to lower elevated blood pressure in overweight and obese persons with high blood pressure. Evidence Category A.

2. Serum/Plasma Lipids

Sixty-five RCT articles were evaluated for the effect of weight loss on serum/plasma concentrations of total cholesterol, LDL-cholesterol, very low-density lipoprotein (VLDL)-cholesterol, triglycerides, and HDL-cholesterol. Studies were conducted on individuals over a range of obesity and lipid levels. Of the 22 articles accepted for inclusion in these guidelines, 14 RCT articles examined lifestyle trials while the remaining 8 articles reviewed pharmacotherapy trials. There is strong evidence from the 14 lifestyle trials that weight loss produced by lifestyle modifications in overweight individuals is accompanied by reductions in serum triglycerides and by increases in HDL-cholesterol. Weight loss generally produces some reductions in serum total cholesterol and LDL-cholesterol. Limited evidence exists that a decrease in abdominal fat correlates with improvements in lipids, although the effect may not be independent of weight loss, and there is strong evidence that increased aerobic activity to increase cardiorespiratory fitness favorably affects blood lipids, particularly if accompanied by weight loss. There is suggestive evidence from the eight randomized pharmacotherapy trials that weight loss produced by weight loss medications and adjuvant lifestyle modifications, including caloric restriction and physical activity, does not result in consistent effects on blood lipids. The following recommendation is based on the review of the data in these 22 RCT articles:

Weight loss is recommended to lower elevated levels of total cholesterol, LDL-cholesterol, and triglycerides, and to raise low levels of HDL-cholesterol in overweight and obese persons with dyslipidemia. Evidence Category A.

3. Blood Glucose

To evaluate the effect of weight loss on fasting blood glucose and fasting insulin levels, 49 RCT articles were reviewed for inclusion in these guidelines. Of the 17 RCT articles accepted, 9 RCT articles examined lifestyle therapy trials and 8 RCT articles considered the effects of pharmacotherapy on weight loss and subsequent changes in blood glucose. There is strong evidence from the nine lifestyle therapy trials that weight loss produced by lifestyle modification reduces blood glucose levels in overweight and obese persons without diabetes, and weight loss reduces blood glucose levels and HbAlc in some patients with type 2 diabetes; there is suggestive evidence that decreases in abdominal fat will improve glucose tolerance in overweight individuals with impaired glucose tolerance, although not independent of weight loss; and there is limited evidence that increased cardiorespiratory fitness improves glucose tolerance in overweight individuals with impaired glucose tolerance or diabetes, although not independent of weight loss. In addition, there is suggestive evidence from randomized trials that weight loss induced by weight loss medications does not appear to improve blood glucose levels any better than weight loss through lifestyle therapy in overweight persons both with and without type 2 diabetes. Based on a full review of the data in these 17 RCT articles, the panel makes the following recommendation:

Weight loss is recommended to lower elevated blood glucose levels in overweight and obese persons with type 2 diabetes. Evidence Category A.

B. Measurement of Degree of Overweight And Obesity

Patients should have their BMI and levels of abdominal fat measured not only for the initial assessment of the degree of overweight and obesity, but also as a guide to the efficacy of weight loss treatment. Although there are no RCTs that review measurements of overweight and obesity, the panel determined that this aspect of patient care warranted further consideration and that this guidance was deemed valuable. Therefore, the following four recommendations that are included in the Treatment Guidelines were based on nonrandomized studies as well as clinical experience.

1. BMI To Assess Overweight and Obesity

There are a number of accurate methods to assess body fat (e.g., total body water, total body potassium, bioelectrical impedance, and dual-energy X-ray absorptiometry), but no trial data exist to indicate that one measure of fatness is better than any other for following overweight and obese patients during treatment. Since measuring body fat by these techniques is often expensive and is not readily available, a more practical approach for the clinical setting is the measurement of BMI; epidemiological and observational studies have shown that BMI provides an acceptable approximation of total body fat for the majority of patients. Because there are no published studies that compare the effectiveness of different measures for evaluating changes in body fat during weight reduction, the panel bases its recommendation on expert judgment from clinical experience:

Practitioners should use the BMI to assess overweight and obesity. Body weight alone can be used to follow weight loss, and to determine efficacy of therapy. Evidence Category C.

2. BMI To Estimate Relative Risk

In epidemiological studies, BMI is the favored measure of excess weight to estimate relative risk of disease. BMI correlates both with morbidity and mortality; the relative risk for CVD [cardiovascular disease] risk factors and CVD incidence increases in a graded fashion with increasing BMI in all population groups. Moreover, calculating BMI is simple, rapid, and inexpensive, and can be applied generally to adults. The panel, therefore, makes this recommendation:

The BMI should be used to classify overweight and obesity and to estimate relative risk of disease compared to normal weight. Evidence Category C.

3. Assessing Abdominal Fat

For the most effective technique for assessing abdominal fat content, the panel considered measures of waist circumference, waist-to-hip ratio (WHR), magnetic resonance imaging (MRI), and computed tomography. Evidence from epidemiological studies shows waist circumference to be a better marker of abdominal fat content than WHR, and that it is the most practical anthropometric measurement for assessing a patient's abdominal fat content before and during weight loss treatment. Computed tomography and MRI are both more accurate but impractical for routine clinical use. Based on evidence that waist circumference is a better marker than WHR—and taking into account that the MRI and computed tomography techniques are expensive and not readily available for clinical practice—the panel makes the following recommendation:

The waist circumference should be used to assess abdominal fat content. Evidence Category C.

4. Sex-Specific Measurements

Evidence from epidemiological studies indicates that a high waist circumference is associated with an increased risk for type 2 diabetes, dyslipidemia, hypertension, and CVD. Therefore, the panel judged that sex-specific cutoffs for waist circumference can be used to identify increased risk associated with abdominal fat in adults with a BMI in the range of 25 to 34.9. These cutpoints can be applied to all adult ethnic or racial groups. On the other hand, if a patient is very short, or has a BMI above the 25 to 34.9 range, waist cutpoints used for the general population may not be applicable. Based on the evidence from nonrandomized studies, the panel makes this recommendation:

For adult patients with a BMI of 25 to 34.9 kg/m^2, sex-specific waist circumference cutoffs should be used in conjunction with BMI to identify increased disease risks. Evidence Category C.

C. Goals for Weight Loss

The general goals of weight loss and management are to reduce body weight, to maintain a lower body weight over the long term, and to prevent further weight gain. Evidence indicates that a moderate weight loss can be maintained over time if some form of therapy continues. It is better to maintain a moderate weight loss over a prolonged period than to regain from a marked weight loss.

1. Initial Goal of Weight Loss from Baseline

There is strong and consistent evidence from randomized trials that overweight and obese patients in well-designed programs can achieve a weight loss of as much as 10 percent of baseline weight. In the diet trials, an average of 8 percent of baseline weight was lost. Since this average includes persons who did not lose weight, an individualized goal of 10 percent is reasonable. The panel, therefore, recommends that:

The initial goal of weight loss therapy should be to reduce body weight by approximately 10 percent from baseline. With success, further weight loss can be attempted if indicated through further assessment. Evidence Category A.

2. Amount of Weight Loss

Randomized trials suggest that weight loss at the rate of 1 to 2 lb/week (calorie deficit of 500 to 1,000 kcal/day) commonly occurs for up to 6 months.

Weight loss should be about 1 to 2 lb/week for a period of 6 months, with the subsequent strategy based on the amount of weight lost. Evidence Category B.

D. How To Achieve Weight Loss

The panel reviewed relevant treatment strategies designed for weight loss that can also be used to foster long-term weight control and prevention of weight gain. The consequent recommendations emphasize the potential effectiveness of weight control using multiple interventions and strategies, including dietary therapy, physical activity, behavior therapy, pharmacotherapy, and surgery, as well as combinations of these strategies.

1. Dietary Therapy

The panel reviewed 86 RCT articles to determine the effectiveness of diets on weight loss (including LCDs, very low-calorie diets (VLCDs), vegetarian diets, American Heart Association dietary guidelines, the NCEP's Step I diet with caloric restriction, and other low-fat regimens with varying combinations of macronutrients). Of the 86 articles reviewed, 48 were accepted for inclusion in these guidelines. These RCTs indicate strong and consistent evidence that an average weight loss of 8 percent of initial body weight can be obtained over 3 to 12 months with an LCD and that this weight loss effects a decrease in abdominal fat; and, although lower-fat diets without targeted caloric reduction help promote weight loss by producing a reduced caloric intake, lower-fat diets with targeted caloric reduction promote greater weight loss than lower-fat diets alone. Further, VLCDs produce greater initial weight losses than LCDs (over the long term of >1 year, weight loss is not different than that of the LCDs). In addition, randomized trials suggest that no improvement in cardiorespiratory fitness as measured by VO2 max appears to occur in obese adults who lose weight on LCDs alone without physical activity. The following recommendations are based on the evidence extracted from the 48 accepted articles:

LCDs are recommended for weight loss in overweight and obese persons. Evidence Category A. Reducing fat as part of an LCD is a practical way to reduce calories. Evidence Category A.

Reducing dietary fat alone without reducing calories is not sufficient for weight loss. However, reducing dietary fat, along with reducing dietary carbohydrates, can facilitate caloric reduction. Evidence Category A.

A diet that is individually planned to help create a deficit of 500 to 1,000 kcal/day should be an intregal part of any program aimed at achieving a weight loss of 1 to 2 lb/week. Evidence Category A.

2. Physical Activity

Effects of Physical Activity on Weight Loss

Twenty-three RCT articles were reviewed to determine the effect of physical activity on weight loss, abdominal fat (measured by waist circumference), and changes in cardiorespiratory fitness (VO_2 max). Thirteen of these articles were accepted for inclusion in these guidelines. A review of these articles reveals strong evidence that physical activity alone, i.e., aerobic exercise, in obese adults results in modest weight loss and that physical activity in overweight and obese adults increases cardiorespiratory fitness, independent of weight loss. Randomized trials suggest that increased physical activity in overweight and obese adults reduces abdominal fat only modestly or not at all, and that regular physical activity independently reduces the risk for CVD. The panel's recommendation on physical activity is based on the evidence from these 13 articles:

Physical activity is recommended as part of a comprehensive weight loss therapy and weight control program because it: (1) modestly contributes to weight loss in overweight and obese adults (Evidence Category A), (2) may decrease abdominal fat (Evidence Category B), (3) increases cardiorespiratory fitness (Evidence Category A), and (4) may help with maintenance of weight loss (Evidence Category C).

Physical activity should be an integral part of weight loss therapy and weight maintenance. Initially, moderate levels of physical activity for 30 to 45 minutes, 3 to 5 days a week, should be encouraged. All adults should set a long-term goal to accumulate at least 30 minutes or more of moderate-intensity physical activity on most, and preferably all, days of the week. Evidence Category B.

Effects of Physical Activity and Diet on Weight Loss (Combined Therapy)
Twenty-three RCT articles were reviewed to determine the effects on body weight of a combination of a reduced-calorie diet with increased physical activity. Fifteen of these articles were accepted for inclusion in the guidelines. These articles contain strong evidence that the combination of a reduced-calorie diet and increased physical activity produces greater weight loss than diet alone or physical activity alone, and that the combination of diet and physical activity improves cardiorespiratory fitness as measured by VO_2 max in overweight and obese adults when compared to diet alone. The combined effect of a reduced calorie diet and increased physical activity seemingly produced modestly greater reductions in abdominal fat than either diet alone or physical activity alone, although it has not been shown to be independent of weight loss. The panel's following recommendations are based on the evidence from these articles:

The combination of a reduced calorie diet and increased physical activity is recommended since it produces weight loss that may also result in decreases in abdominal fat and increases in cardiorespiratory fitness. Evidence Category A.

3. Behavior Therapy

Thirty-six RCTs were reviewed to evaluate whether behavior therapy provides additional benefit beyond other weight loss approaches, as well as to compare various behavioral techniques. Of the 36 RCTs reviewed, 22 were accepted. These RCTs strongly indicate that behavioral strategies to reinforce changes in diet and physical activity in obese adults produce weight loss in the range of 10 percent over 4 months to 1 year. In addition, no one behavior therapy appeared superior to any other in its effect on weight loss; multimodal strategies appear to work best and those interventions with the greatest intensity appear to be associated with the greatest weight loss. Long-term follow-up of patients undergoing behavior therapy shows a return to baseline weight for the great majority of subjects in the absence of continued behavioral intervention. Randomized trials suggest that behavior therapy, when used in combination with other weight loss approaches, provides additional benefits in assisting patients to lose weight short-term, i.e., 1 year (no additional benefits are found at 3 to 5 years). The panel found little evidence on the effect of behavior therapy on cardiorespiratory fitness. Evidence from these articles provided the basis for the following recommendation:

Behavior therapy is a useful adjunct when incorporated into treatment for weight loss and weight maintenance. Evidence Category B.

There is also suggestive evidence that patient motivation is a key component for success in a weight loss program. The panel, therefore, makes the following recommendation:

Practitioners need to assess the patient's motivation to enter weight loss therapy; assess the readiness of the patient to implement the plan and then take appropriate steps to motivate the patient for treatment. Evidence Category D.

4. Summary of Lifestyle Therapy

There is strong evidence that combined interventions of an LCD, increased physical activity, and behavior therapy provide the most successful therapy for weight loss and weight maintenance. The panel makes the following recommendation:

Weight loss and weight maintenance therapy should employ the combination of LCD's, increased physical activity, and behavior therapy. Evidence Category A.

5. Pharmacotherapy

A review of 44 pharmacotherapy RCT articles provides strong evidence that pharmacological therapy (which has generally been studied along with lifestyle modification, including diet and physical activity) using dexfenfluramine, sibutramine, orlistat, or phentermine/fenfluramine results in weight loss in obese adults when used for 6 months to 1 year. Strong evidence also indicates that appropriate weight loss drugs can augment diet, physical activity, and behavior therapy in weight loss. Adverse side effects from the use of weight loss drugs have been observed in patients. As a result of the observed association of valvular heart disease in patients taking fenfluramine and dexfenfluramine alone or in combination, these drugs have been withdrawn from the market. Weight loss drugs approved by the FDA [U.S. Food and Drug Administration] for long-term use may be useful as an adjunct to diet and physical activity for patients with a BMI of ≥ 30 with no concomitant obesity-related risk factors or diseases, as well as for patients with a BMI of ≥ 27 with concomitant risk factors or diseases; moreover, using weight loss drugs singly (not in combination) and starting with the lowest effective doses can decrease the likelihood of adverse effects. Based on this evidence, the panel makes the following recommendation:

Weight loss drugs approved by the FDA may be used as part of a comprehensive weight loss program, including dietary therapy and physical activity for patients with a BMI of ≥ 30 with no concomitant obesity-related risk factors or diseases, and for patients with a BMI of ≥ 27 with concomitant obesity-related risk factors or diseases. Weight loss drugs should never be used without concomitant lifestyle modifications. Continual assessment of drug therapy for efficacy and safety is necessary. If the drug is efficacious in helping the patient to lose and/or maintain weight loss and there are no serious adverse effects, it can be continued. If not, it should be discontinued. Evidence Category B.

6. Weight Loss Surgery

The panel reviewed 14 RCTs that examined the effect of surgical procedures on weight loss; 8 were deemed appropriate. All of the studies included individuals who had a BMI of 40 kg/m^2 or above, or a BMI of 35 to 40 kg/m^2 with comorbidity. These trials provide strong evidence that surgical interventions in adults with clinically severe obesity, i.e., BMIs ≥40 or ≥35 with comorbid conditions, result in substantial weight loss, and suggestive evidence that lifelong medical surveillance after surgery is necessary. Therefore, the panel makes the following recommendation:

Weight loss surgery is an option for carefully selected patients with clinically severe obesity (BMI ≥40 or ≥35 with co-morbid conditions) when less invasive methods of weight loss have failed and the patient is at high risk for obesity-associated morbidity or mortality. Evidence Category B.

E. Goals For Weight Loss Maintenance

Once the goals of weight loss have been successfully achieved, maintenance of a lower body weight becomes the challenge. Whereas studies have shown that weight loss is achievable, it is difficult to maintain over a long period of time (3 to 5 years). In fact, the majority of persons who lose weight, once dismissed from clinical therapy, frequently regain it —so the challenge to the patient and the practitioner is to maintain the weight loss. Successful weight reduction thus depends on continuing a maintenance program on a long-term basis. In the past, obtaining the goal of weight loss has been considered the end of weight loss therapy. Observation, monitoring, and encouragement of patients who have successfully lost weight should be continued long term. The panel's recommendations on weight loss maintenance are derived from RCT evidence as well as nonrandomized and observational studies.

1. Weight Maintenance Phase

RCTs from the Behavior Therapy section above suggest that lost weight usually will be regained unless a weight maintenance program consisting of dietary therapy, physical activity, and behavior therapy is continued indefinitely. Drug therapy in addition may be helpful during the weight maintenance phase. The panel also reviewed RCT evidence that considered the rate of weight loss and the role of weight maintenance. These RCTs suggest that after 6 months of weight loss treatment, efforts to maintain weight loss are important. Therefore, the panel recommends the following:

After successful weight loss, the likelihood of weight loss maintenance is enhanced by a program consisting of dietary therapy, physical activity, and behavior therapy which should be continued indefinitely. Drug therapy can also be used. However, drug safety and efficacy beyond 1 year of total treatment have not been established. Evidence Category B.

A weight maintenance program should be a priority after the initial 6 months of weight loss therapy. Evidence Category B.

Strong evidence indicates that better weight loss results are achieved with dietary therapy when the duration of the intervention is at least 6 months. Suggestive evidence also indicates that during dietary therapy, frequent contacts between professional counselors and patients promote weight loss and maintenance. Therefore, the panel recommends the following:

> *The literature suggests that weight loss and weight maintenance therapies that provide a grater frequency of contacts between the patient and the practitioner and are provided over the long term should be utilized whenever possible. This can lead to more successful weight loss and weight maintenance. Evidence Category C.*

> Source: National Heart, Blood and Lung Institute. "Executive Summary." In *Clinical Guidelines on the Identification, Evaluation, and Treatment of Overweight and Obesity in Adults* NIH Publication No. 98-4083. Bethesda, MD: U.S. Department of Health and Human Services, 1998, xxi–xxix.

"The Surgeon General's Call to Action to Prevent and Decrease Overweight and Obesity"

On December 13, 2001, U.S. Surgeon General David Satcher declared that the nationwide rise inoverweight and obesity was a major public health issue facing the United States. The surgeon general's report emphasized the magnitude of the concern by drawing on statistical data showing the rising trend in obesity and overweight in the United States and documenting the associated health risks and economic impact. In the Foreward, Dr. Satcher states, "Many people believe that dealing with overweight and obesity is a personal responsibility. To some degree they are right, but it is also a community responsibility" (p. xiii).

Satcher acknowledged that no clear evidence was available to determine how to effectively prevent and reduce obesity and overweight. He reasoned that this lack of information demanded a concerted national public health response. The "Call to Action" urged a cooperative effort from individuals, families, communities, schools, work sites, organizations, and the media to find new ways to reduce and prevent overweight and obesity. The goal of the "Call to Action" is to set priorities, establish strategies and actions at multiple levels, and provide a starting point for groups and individuals to address this national health problem.

In preparing the report, the Surgeon General's Office held a public comment period to gather ideas from clinicians, researchers, consumers, and advocates. The sessions generated numerous community-based strategies that were organized into five key settings: families and communities, schools, health care, media and communications, and work sites. Interventions for the settings were further grouped into categories of communication, action, research, and evaluation (CARE).

Two excerpts are shown here. The first is a statement of principles established to help meet these new public health objectives, and the second is a portion from Section 2 that provides an example of how the CARE framework was used to develop public health programs and implement strategic actions that may reduce overweight and obesity in the United States.

The Surgeon General's Call To Action To Prevent and Decrease Overweight and Obesity

Principles:

Overweight and obesity have reached nationwide epidemic proportions. Both the prevention and treatment of overweight and obesity and their associated health problems are important public health goals. To achieve these goals, the *Surgeon General's Call To Action To Prevent and Decrease Overweight and Obesity* is committed to five overarching principles:

1. Promote the recognition of overweight and obesity as major public health problems.
2. Assist Americans in balancing healthful eating with regular physical activity to achieve and maintain a healthy or healthier body weight.
3. Identify effective and culturally appropriate interventions to prevent and treat overweight and obesity.
4. Encourage environmental changes that help prevent overweight and obesity.
5. Develop and enhance public-private partnerships to help implement this vision.

Section 2. Posing Questions and Developing Strategies
Developing a Public Health Response
CARE To Address Overweight and Obesity

Current knowledge is clear on many issues: the prevalence of overweight and obesity is high, and that of obesity is increasing rapidly;

adolescents who are overweight are at high risk of becoming overweight or obese adults; overweight and obesity increase the risk for serious diseases such as type 2 diabetes, hypertension, and high blood cholesterol; and overweight and obesity are associated with premature death and disability. It is also known that a healthy diet and adequate physical activity aid in maintaining a healthy weight and, among overweight or obese persons, can promote weight loss. Knowledge is less clear, however, on some very important questions. How can overweight and obesity be prevented? What are the most effective prevention and treatment strategies? How can the environment be modified to promote healthier eating and increased physical activity? Determining the answers to these questions demands a national public health response. Assembling the components of this response has begun.

Developing a Public Health Response

In December 2000, the Surgeon General hosted a public Listening Session on overweight and obesity. The meeting—Toward a National Action Plan on Overweight and Obesity: The Surgeon General's Initiative—began a developmental process that led to this *Surgeon General's Call To Action To Prevent and Decrease Overweight and Obesity*. A menu of important activities has been assembled from comments received during the Surgeon General's Listening Session, a public comment period, and the National Nutrition Summit. The menu, which is presented in the following section, highlights areas that received significant attention during one or more of these events. Although not meant to be prescriptive, the menu should establish useful starting points as individuals and groups focus their own skills, creativity, and inspiration on the national epidemic of overweight and obesity.

The discussions at the Surgeon General's Listening Session centered on activities and interventions in five key settings: families and communities, schools, health care, media and communications, and worksites. The key actions discussed are presented for each of these settings. Many of these actions overlap the different settings and can be applied in several or all environments.

CARE To Address Overweight and Obesity

The key actions are organized by setting in a framework called CARE: Communication, Action, and Research and Evaluation.

Communication: Provision of information and tools to motivate and empower decision makers at the governmental, organizational, community, family, and individual levels who will create change toward the prevention and decrease of overweight and obesity.

Action: Interventions and activities that assist decision makers in preventing and decreasing overweight and obesity, individually or collectively.

Research and Evaluation: Investigations to better understand the causes of overweight and obesity, to assess the effectiveness of interventions, and to develop new communication and action strategies. Within the CARE framework, effective actions must occur at multiple levels. Obviously, individual behavioral change lies at the core of all strategies to reduce overweight and obesity. Successful efforts, however, must focus not only on individual behavioral change, but also on group influences, institutional and community influences, and public policy. Actions to reduce overweight and obesity will fail without this multidimensional approach. Individual behavioral change can occur only in a supportive environment with accessible and affordable healthy food choices and opportunities for regular physical activity. Furthermore, actions aimed exclusively at individual behavioral change, while not considering social, cultural, economic, and environmental influences, are likely to reinforce attitudes of stigmatization against the overweight and obese.

Setting 1: Families and Communities

Families and communities lie at the foundation of the solution to the problems of overweight and obesity. Family members can share their own knowledge and habits regarding a healthy diet and physical activity with their children, friends, and other community members. Emphasis should be placed on family and community opportunities for communication, education, and peer support surrounding the maintenance of healthy dietary choices and physical activity patterns.

Communication

1. Raise consumer awareness about the effect of being overweight on overall health.
2. Inform community leaders about the importance of developing healthy communities.
3. Highlight programs that support healthful food and physical activity choices to community decision makers.
4. Raise policy makers' awareness of the need to develop social and environmental policy that would help communities and families be more physically active and consume a healthier diet.
5. Educate individuals, families, and communities about healthy dietary patterns and regular physical activity, based on the *Dietary Guidelines for Americans*.

6. Educate parents about the need to serve as good role models by practicing healthy eating habits and engaging in regular physical activity in order to instill lifelong healthy habits in their children.
7. Raise consumer awareness about reasonable food and beverage portion sizes.
8. Educate expectant parents and other community members about the potentially protective effect of breast-feeding against the development of obesity.

Action

1. Form community coalitions to support the development of increased opportunities to engage in leisure time physical activity and to encourage food outlets to increase availability of low-calorie, nutritious food items.
2. Encourage the food industry to provide reasonable food and beverage portion sizes.
3. Increase availability of nutrition information for foods eaten and prepared away from home.
4. Create more community-based obesity prevention and treatment programs for children and adults.
5. Empower families to manage weight and health through skill building in parenting, meal planning, and behavioral management.
6. Expand efforts to encourage healthy eating patterns, consistent with the *Dietary Guidelines for Americans*, by nutrition assistance recipients.
7. Provide demonstration grants to address the lack of access to and availability of healthy affordable foods in inner cities.
8. Promote healthful dietary patterns, including consumption of at least five servings of fruits and vegetables a day.
9. Create community environments that promote and support breastfeeding.
10. Decrease time spent watching television and in similar sedentary behaviors by children and their families.
11. Provide demonstration grants to address the lack of public access to safe and supervised physical activity.

12. Create and implement public policy related to the provision of safe and accessible sidewalks, walking and bicycle paths, and stairs.

Research and Evaluation

1. Conduct research on obesity prevention and reduction to confirm their effects on improving health outcomes.
2. Determine the root causes, behaviors, and social and ecological factors leading to obesity and how such forces vary by race and ethnicity, gender, and socioeconomic status.
3. Assess the factors contributing to the disproportionate burden of overweight and obesity in low-income and minority racial and ethnic populations.
4. Develop and evaluate preventive interventions that target infants and children, especially those who are at high risk of becoming obese.
5. Coordinate research activities to refine risk assessment, to enhance obesity prevention, and to support appropriate consumer messages and education.
6. Study the cost-effectiveness of community-directed strategies designed to prevent the onset of overweight and obesity.
7. Conduct behavioral research to identify how to motivate people to increase and maintain physical activity and make healthier food choices.
8. Evaluate the feasibility of incentives that support healthful dietary and physical activity patterns.
9. Identify techniques that can foster community motivation to reduce overweight and obesity.
10. Examine the marketing practices of the fast food industry and the factors determining construction of new food outlets.

Setting 2: Schools

Schools are identified as a key setting for public health strategies to prevent and decrease the prevalence of overweight and obesity. Most children spend a large portion of time in school. Schools provide many opportunities to engage children in healthy eating and physical activity and to reinforce healthy diet and physical activity messages. Public health approaches in schools should extend beyond health and physical education to include school policy, the school physical and social environment, and links between schools and families and communities. Schools and communities that are interested in reducing overweight among the young people they serve can consider options listed below. Decisions about which options to select should be made at the local level.

Communication

1. Build awareness among teachers, food service staff, coaches, nurses, and other school staff about the contribution of proper nutrition and physical activity to the maintenance of lifelong healthy weight.
2. Educate teachers, staff, and parents about the importance of school physical activity and nutrition programs and policies.
3. Educate parents, teachers, coaches, staff, and other adults in the community about the importance they hold as role models for children, and teach them how to be models for healthy eating and regular physical activity.
4. Educate students, teachers, staff, and parents about the importance of body size acceptance and the dangers of unhealthy weight control practices.
5. Develop sensitivity of staff to the problems encountered by the overweight child.

Action

1. Provide age-appropriate and culturally sensitive instruction in health education that helps students develop the knowledge, attitudes, skills, and behaviors to adopt, maintain, and enjoy healthy eating habits and a physically active lifestyle.
2. Ensure that meals offered through the school breakfast and lunch programs meet nutrition standards.
3. Adopt policies ensuring that all foods and beverages available on school campuses and at school events contribute toward eating patterns that are consistent with the *Dietary Guidelines for Americans*.
4. Provide food options that are low in fat, calories, and added sugars, such as fruits, vegetables, whole grains, and low-fat or nonfat dairy foods.

5. Ensure that healthy snacks and foods are provided in vending machines, school stores, and other venues within the school's control.
6. Prohibit student access to vending machines, school stores, and other venues that compete with healthy school meals in elementary schools and restrict access in middle, junior, and high schools.
7. Provide an adequate amount of time for students to eat school meals, and schedule lunch periods at reasonable hours around midday.
8. Provide all children, from prekindergarten through grade 12, with quality daily physical education that helps develop the knowledge, attitudes, skills, behaviors, and confidence needed to be physically active for life.
9. Provide daily recess periods for elementary school students, featuring time for unstructured but supervised play.
10. Provide extracurricular physical activity programs, especially inclusive intramural programs and physical activity clubs.
11. Encourage the use of school facilities for physical activity programs offered by the school and/or community-based organizations outside of school hours.

Research and Evaluation

1. Conduct research on the relationship of healthy eating and physical activity to student health, learning, attendance, classroom behavior, violence, and other social outcomes.
2. Evaluate school-based behavioral health interventions for the prevention of overweight in children.
3. Develop an ongoing, systematic process to assess the school physical activity and nutrition environment, and plan, implement, and monitor improvements.
4. Conduct research to study the effect of school policies such as food services and physical activity curricula on overweight in children and adolescents.
5. Evaluate the financial and health impact of school contracts with vendors of high- calorie foods and beverages with minimal nutritional value.

Setting 3: Health Care

The health care system provides a powerful setting for interventions aimed at reducing the prevalence of overweight and obesity and their consequences. A majority of Americans interact with the health care system at least once during any given year. Recommendations by pediatric and adult health care providers can be influential in patient dietary choices and physical activity patterns. In collaboration with schools and worksites, health care providers and institutions can reinforce the adoption and maintenance of healthy lifestyle behaviors. Health care providers also can serve as effective public policy advocates and further catalyze intervention efforts in the family and the community and in the media communications settings.

Communication

1. Inform health care providers and administrators of the tremendous burden of overweight and obesity on the health care system in terms of mortality, morbidity, and cost.
2. Inform and educate the health care community about the importance of healthy eating, consistent with the *Dietary Guidelines for Americans,* and physical activity and fitness for the promotion of health.
3. Educate health care providers and administrators to identify and reduce the barriers involving patients' lack of access to effective nutrition and physical activity interventions.
4. Inform and educate the health care community about assessment of weight status and the risk of inappropriate weight change.
5. Educate health care providers on effective ways to promote and support breastfeeding.

Action

1. Train health care providers and health profession students in effective prevention and treatment techniques for overweight and obesity.
2. Encourage partnerships between health care providers, schools, faith-based groups, and other community organizations in prevention efforts targeted at social and environmental causes of overweight and obesity.

3. Establish a dialogue to consider classifying obesity as a disease category for reimbursement coding.
4. Explore mechanisms that will partially or fully cover reimbursement or include as a member benefit health care services associated with weight management, including nutrition education and physical activity programs.

Research and Evaluation

1. Develop effective preventive and therapeutic programs for obesity.
2. Study the effect of weight reduction programs on health outcomes.
3. Analyze the cost-effectiveness data on clinical obesity prevention and treatment efforts and conduct further research where the data are inconclusive.
4. Promote research on the maintenance of weight loss.
5. Promote research on breastfeeding and the prevention of obesity.
6. Review and evaluate the reimbursement policies of public and private health insurance providers regarding overweight and obesity prevention and treatment efforts.

Setting 4: Media and Communications

The media can provide essential functions in overweight and obesity prevention efforts. From a public education and social marketing standpoint, the media can disseminate health messages and display healthy behaviors aimed at changing dietary habits and exercise patterns. In addition, the media can provide a powerful forum for community members who are addressing the social and environmental influences on dietary and physical activity patterns.

Communication

1. Emphasize to media professionals that the primary concern of overweight and obesity is one of health rather than appearance.
2. Emphasize to media professionals the disproportionate burden of overweight and obesity in low-income and

racial and ethnic minority populations and the need for culturally sensitive health messages.

3. Communicate the importance of prevention of overweight through balancing food intake with physical activity at all ages.
4. Promote the recognition of inappropriate weight change.
5. Build awareness of the importance of social and environmental influences on making appropriate diet and physical activity choices.
6. Provide professional education for media professionals on policy areas related to diet and physical activity.
7. Emphasize to media professionals the need to develop uniform health messages about physical activity and nutrition that are consistent with the *Dietary Guidelines for Americans.*

Action

1. Conduct a national campaign to foster public awareness of the health benefits of regular physical activity, healthful dietary choices, and maintaining a healthy weight, based on the *Dietary Guidelines for Americans.*
2. Encourage truthful and reasonable consumer goals for weight loss programs and weight management products.
3. Incorporate messages about proper nutrition, including eating at least five servings of fruits and vegetables a day, and regular physical activity in youth-oriented TV programming.
4. Train nutrition and exercise scientists and specialists in media advocacy skills that will empower them to disseminate their knowledge to a broad audience.
5. Encourage community-based advertising campaigns to balance messages that may encourage consumption of excess calories and inactivity generated by fast food industries and by industries that promote sedentary behaviors.
6. Encourage media professionals to utilize actors' influences as role models to demonstrate eating and physical activity lifestyles for health rather than for appearance.
7. Encourage media professionals to employ actors of diverse sizes.

Research and Evaluation

1. Evaluate the impact of community media advocacy campaigns designed to achieve public policy and health-related goals.
2. Conduct consumer research to ensure that media messages are positive, realistic, relevant, consistent, and achievable.
3. Increase research on the effects of popular media images of ideal body types and their potential health impact, particularly on young women.

Setting 5: Worksites

More than 100 million Americans spend the majority of their day at a worksite. While at work, employees are often aggregated within systems for communication, education, and peer support. Thus, worksites provide many opportunities to reinforce the adoption and maintenance of healthy lifestyle behaviors. Public health approaches in worksites should extend beyond health education and awareness to include worksite policies, the physical and social environments of worksites, and their links with the family and community setting.

Communication

1. Inform employers of the direct and indirect costs of obesity.
2. Communicate to employers the return-on-investment (ROI) data for worksite obesity prevention and treatment strategies.

Action

1. Change workflow patterns, including flexible work hours, to create opportunities for regular physical activity during the workday.
2. Provide protected time for lunch, and ensure that healthy food options are available.
3. Establish worksite exercise facilities or create incentives for employees to join local fitness centers.
4. Create incentives for workers to achieve and maintain a healthy body weight.

5. Encourage employers to require weight management and physical activity counseling as a member benefit in health insurance contracts.
6. Create work environments that promote and support breastfeeding.
7. Explore ways to create Federal worksite programs promoting healthy eating and physical activity that will set an example to the private sector.

Research and Evaluation

1. Evaluate best practices in worksite overweight and obesity prevention and treatment efforts, and disseminate results of studies widely.
2. Evaluate economic data examining worksite obesity prevention and treatment efforts.
3. Conduct controlled worksite studies of the impact of overweight and obesity management programs on worker productivity and absenteeism.

Source: U.S. Department of Health and Human Services.
"The Surgeon General's Call to Action to
Prevent and Decrease Overweight and Obesity."
Rockville, MD: Office of the Surgeon General, 2001.
Principles v; Section 2. Posing Questions and Developing Strategies 15–24.

Strategic Plan for NIH Obesity Research

The U.S. National Institutes of Health (NIH) supports research that provides a scientific evidence base for public policy decisions.The NIH) invests more than $28 billion annually in medical research and is the primary federal agency for conducting and supporting medical research. It consists of 27 institutes and centers and provides direction and financial support through competitive grants to researchers in the United States and throughout the world. Currently, the NIH funds more than 90 percent of all obesity research in the United States.

Obesity research is by nature multidisciplinary, involving a broad range of studies, including molecular, genetic, behavioral, environmental, clinical, and epidemiologic investigations. In light of this diversity, Elias A. Zerhouni, MD, director of the NIH, created the NIH Obesity Research Task Force to intensify basic and clinical research and to help coordinate obesity research across the NIH's institutes and centers. In 2004, the Task Force developed and published theStrategic Plan for

NIH Obesity Research. The plan is a guide for supporting innovative and collaborative research in a comprehensive way.

The plan's obesity research goals range from identification of the underlying causes to potential behavioral, pharmacologic, and surgical treatments to reduction of associated diseases to translation of basic science results into useful advice for the public. The excerpt illustrates the diversity and collaboration in ongoing NIH research efforts, with examples related to the development of clinical nutrition research units (CNRUs), methods of health behavior surveillance, the effectiveness of low- and high-carbohydrate diets and bariatric surgery, and the creation of new, standardized mouse models to help study obesity.

Strategic Plan for NIH Obesity Research
Appendix B: Examples of Ongoing
NIH Efforts

Introduction

This Appendix highlights examples of ongoing NIH efforts relevant to obesity research. These efforts are among the strategies and opportunities supported by the NIH to achieve its goals for: research toward preventing and treating obesity through lifestyle modification; research toward preventing and treating obesity through pharmacologic, surgical, or other medical approaches; research toward breaking the link between obesity and its associated health conditions; and cross-cutting research topics, including technologies, fostering of multidisciplinary and interdisciplinary research teams, investigator training, translational research and education/ outreach efforts.

Clinical Nutrition Research Units (CNRUs) and Obesity/Nutrition Research Centers (ONRCs):
The CNRU/ONRC program provides important resources for the obesity research community. There are ten CNRUs and four ONRCs, located throughout the country. These Centers are integrated arrays of research, shared resources, educational, clinical, and training opportunities. These Centers pursue basic and clinical research, including such cross-cutting areas as multidisciplinary research and translational research, and offer a rich environment for research training related to obesity and nutritional sciences.

Advances in obesity research are derived from such fundamental disciplines as biochemistry, molecular biology, genetics, and physiology; and such medical specialties as internal medicine, pediatrics, and surgery. Because of its interdisciplinary nature, obesity research can benefit from close interactions among researchers; health services providers, and educators. Supported by the NIH, the core centers for shared research facilities at CNRUs and ONRCs are a valuable way to promote multidisciplinary interactions, fostering and strengthening obesity research within a broad nutritional science context.

The CNRUs and ONRCs conduct research on treatment and prevention of obesity and eating disorders, understanding of the control and modulation of energy metabolism as related to obesity, and understanding and treatment of other health conditions associated with abnormalities of energy balance and weight management. As one objective, these Centers strive to promote basic and clinical science studies to advance understanding of the complex interrelationships among genetic factors and the environment in obesity and other health conditions, such as diabetes, cardiovascular disease, and cancer. The CNRUs/ONRCs are poised to stimulate and support development and use of state-of-the-art techniques to study nutritional factors and their influence on these and other health conditions. Another objective of the Centers is to encourage translational studies that apply newer basic science findings to the diagnosis and management of obesity and other chronic health conditions.

All CNRUs and ONRCs are required to conduct clinical studies. The clinical investigation component facilitates translation of research into practical treatment strategies for patients, provides Center investigators with clinical samples and patient data needed for their research, and serves as a bridge between clinical and basic science investigators. Most of the Centers have a clinic population with adequate representation of women and minorities who can readily participate in research studies. The availability of such a population plays a major role in attracting investigators to the field of obesity research, and also can facilitate the design of pilot and feasibility projects (discussed below). The emphasis on clinical research in the CNRUs and ONRCs further provides a natural interaction with the NIH-supported General Clinical Research Centers (GCRCs). The GCRCs are an additional resource for experimental design and instrumentation to advance the pursuit of pathophysiological mechanisms of obesity-related diseases in humans.

Another valuable aspect of the CNRUs and ONRCs is an associated pilot and feasibility program. This program provides support for new investigators or for established investigators who are moving into areas of research relevant to the goals of the Centers. Projects evaluating the effectiveness of model programs for translating research in biomedical and behavioral science into routine clinical care also are encouraged. The combination of the shared core resources, clinical research expertise, and support for pilot and feasibility studies also permits the CNRUs and ONRCs a way to move quickly to study "natural experiments." For example, protocols could be designed to assess the efficacy of proposed policy changes in schools concerning food offerings and/or physical activity, or to study obesity-focused efforts of food companies or restaurants.

Finally, many of the CNRUs/ONRCs are co-located at institutions with Schools of Public Health and CDC [Centers for Disease Control and Prevention]-supported Prevention Centers. Thus, these locations should be primed to respond to new initiatives, especially those targeting prevention at the community and population level.

Preventing and Treating Obesity Through Behavioral and Environmental Approaches To Modify Lifestyle

Environmental approaches to obesity prevention:
As a result of a recently launched NIH initiative in this area, a variety of new studies are now under way to develop and test environmental modifications aimed toward preventing obesity in children as well as adults. Environments targeted by these studies that are relevant to children include, for example, child care centers, schools, after-school programs, and the home; studies relevant to adults include, for example, a cafeteria-based study based in a community center. In addition to designing interventions to be tested, two of the projects will be "natural experiments" to evaluate the impact on health outcomes of new school policies, developed by policy-makers in Seattle and California that relate to commercial advertising, the sale of energy-dense foods, and other issues. Among the studies being supported as a result of this initiative, some have a particular focus on minority populations disproportionately affected by obesity, including African Americans and American Indians.

Diabetes Prevention Program Outcome Study (DPPOS):
A follow-up study of participants in the DPP clinical trial (described previously) will examine the durability of the DPP interventions on prevention or delay of type 2 diabetes and its cardiovascular complications; heart disease is the major cause of death in people with type 2 diabetes. The DPPOS will additionally examine the ability to maintain weight loss in the participants over extended periods of time.

Look AHEAD (Action for Health in Diabetes) clinical trial:
This multi-center, NIH-sponsored clinical trial will examine the health effects of an intervention designed to achieve and maintain weight loss over the long term through decreased caloric intake and increased physical activity. Look AHEAD has a goal of enrolling 5,000 obese patients with type 2 diabetes, including both men and women and members of minority groups, and following them for up to 11.5 years to study the impact of the weight loss intervention on cardiovascular disease, the complication of diabetes that causes the greatest rates of illness and death.

National Health and Nutrition Examination Survey (NHANES):
The NIH provides additional resources to NHANES, a series of surveys conducted by the National Center for Health Statistics of the CDC.

The goals of NHANES include estimating the number of people in the U.S. who have selected diseases, analyzing risk factors for diseases, and studying the relationship between diet, nutrition, physical activity, and health. Measurement of body composition and cardiorespiratory fitness are two of the components of NHANES currently supported by the NIH. The body composition measure will provide information on fat mass and percent body fat for the U.S. population, and the cardiorespiratory fitness measure will provide information on fitness for those ages 12 to 49 years. These data provide detail beyond body mass index and reported physical activity to be linked with other important health status and public health information.

In addition, the NIH has supported improvements in the methods for assessing diet and physical activity, including the addition of an objective measure of physical activity—key elements for understanding population targets for interventions to prevent and treat obesity. The NIH will also explore the potential of supporting a longitudinal component to NHANES to examine changes in weight over the lifetime in diverse population groups.

National and regional surveillance of health behaviors:
The NIH provides support for cancer control supplements and other data elements within the National Health Interview Survey and the California Health Interview Survey. These surveys result in representative data concerning diverse health behaviors, including diet and physical activity.

Current NIH efforts are focusing on using these surveys to better understand disparities in levels of physical activity among different race/ethnic groups and to develop capacity for analyzing associations between the environment and physical activity. Such efforts complement data from NHANES because they provide larger samples for specific racial and ethnic groups at high risk for obesity and more extensive coverage of regional and state diversity in obesity related health behaviors.

Weight-loss maintenance:
Because maintenance of weight loss is a critical yet particularly difficult element of obesity treatment and prevention, the newly launched Weight Loss Maintenance Trial will compare different strategies for maintaining weight loss over a period of 2 1/2 years in approximately 800 adults who are at high risk for cardiovascular disease and who are successful in losing a targeted amount of weight over the short term through lifestyle changes.

Long-term evaluation of factors associated with childhood obesity or its associated health problems:
Investigators in the intramural program at NIH are conducting a longitudinal study in which 250 children who are either overweight or at risk for overweight are extensively evaluated for factors that may predict

development of obesity or its associated health conditions, including genetic variation, metabolic and cardiovascular differences, food intake, total and resting energy expenditure, psychological functioning, eating disorders, and physical activity behaviors. These children are being followed for 15 years, and should provide valuable information on risks for the development of obesity and its medical complications.

The Girls Health Enrichment Multi-site Studies (GEMS):
This research effort is a two-phase program to develop and pilot-test interventions to prevent obesity in African American girls ages 8 to 10 years, a group at high risk of developing obesity. During Phase 1, several distinct interventions addressing diet, physical activity, and psychosocial and family influences were developed and pilot tested. During Phase 2, two field centers are testing separate 2-year interventions to reduce excessive weight gain in African American girls ages 8–10 years. One study is testing a family-based program that counsels and teaches 300 girls and their parents or caregivers to eat healthy diets, drink fewer sweetened beverages, and increase their physical activity. The second study of 260 girls is testing an intervention that encourages girls to attend after-school dance classes set up in the community to increase their physical activity and also delivers a home-based intervention to reduce girls' TV watching to reduce the amount of time they are sedentary and exposed to food advertising and eating opportunities.

The PREMIER trial—to determine the effectiveness of multicomponent lifestyle intervention programs in lowering blood pressure:
A total of 810 participants were randomly assigned to receive one of 3 interventions over an 18 month period: 1) an intensive behavioral intervention to facilitate their achieving lifestyle changes that are currently recommended for blood pressure control—reduced salt intake, increased physical activity, and weight control or weight loss, as needed; 2) this same intervention coupled with a behavioral intervention to promote consumption of the DASH [Dietary Approaches to Stop Hypertension] diet (an eating pattern rich in fruits, vegetables, and low fat dairy products; low in total and saturated fat and cholesterol; and moderately high in protein), which has been shown to lower blood pressure; or 3) advice alone.

The Dietary Composition, Obesity, and Cardiovascular Risk study:
This study investigates the effects of energy density and three different macronutrient (protein, fat, carbohydrate) compositions of diet on coronary heart disease risk factors (LDL-cholesterol, HDL-cholesterol, remnant lipoprotein c, Lp(a) cholesterol, insulin, glycosylated hemoglobin, glucose, and blood pressure) in the fasting and nonfasting state (4 hours after a meal) in 80 men and women (men ages 50 to 67 years and postmenopausal women under 65 years) with elevated LDL-cholesterol (130 mg/dL or greater) and overweight or obese (BMI 28–38 kg/m^2). A

12-week controlled diet feeding study followed by participants' preparing their own foods on their assigned diets for 1 year investigates the effects of energy density and various macronutrient composition (calories, fat, protein, carbohydrate, and dietary glycemic index) on energy balance and cardiovascular disease risk factors such as body weight and composition, physical activity, blood pressure, and plasma lipoproteins. This study plans to find out whether diets low in caloric density, regardless of overall fat intake or glycemic index, will have a more favorable effect on coronary heart disease risk factors, body weight and composition, and energy expenditure than a diet with higher caloric density and high glycemic index.

Dietary Macronutrients and Weight Loss:
This trial investigates whether the macronutrient composition of the diet (the relative amount of fat, protein, and carbohydrate) can help promote weight loss and its maintenance. The trial compares the effects on weight loss and weight maintenance of four diets differing in macronutrient composition in 800 overweight or obese adults over a two-year period. The diets are all low in saturated fat. The four diets are a moderate fat diet and a low fat diet, each at two levels of protein. Participants are counseled to follow these diets using a state-of-the art behavioral program.

Low and high carbohydrate diets:
The Safety and Efficacy of Low and High Carbohydrate Diets study is assessing the short-term and long-term clinical effects of different diets in 360 obese men and women.

Participants in a 26-week behavioral weight loss program will be randomized to a diet featuring low carbohydrate, unlimited fat and protein, or to a conventional diet of high carbohydrate and low fat. Short-term (weeks 12–26) and long-term (weeks 52–104) effects of each dietary approach will be evaluated and compared in terms of changes in weight and body composition, metabolic and organ function, and exercise endurance.

Behavioral Change Consortium:
This initiative was designed to stimulate investigations of innovative strategies designed to achieve long-term healthy behavior change. A large number of the funded projects are focusing specifically on physical activity and/or dietary behaviors. These projects include

The SENIOR Project; Youth Environments Promoting Nutrition and Activity; Promoting Healthy Lifestyles: Alternative Models' Effects; Project HOPE; Exercise Advice by Human or Computer; Reducing Disease Risk in Low-income, Postpartum Women; and Health Promotion Through Black Churches. In addition, consortia working groups in nutrition and physical activity have been established to coordinate cross-site analyses of common research measures.

Maintenance of long-term behavior change:
As a result of another NIH effort, new research is beginning on the biopsychosocial processes and interventions that target long-term maintenance of behavior change, including behavior relevant to overweight and obesity such as physical activity.

Obesity and the built environment—improving public health through community design:
The built environment encompasses all of the buildings, spaces, and products created or modified by people, including, for example: buildings (housing, schools, workplaces), land use (industrial or residential), public resources (parks, museums), zoning regulations, and transportation systems. An NIH-sponsored conference was held to provide a forum to discuss how different elements of the built environment may contribute to obesity via access to food and physical activity, and how environmental health research and interventions could address this public health problem. The goals of the conference included developing research and practice agendas to examine the relationship between the built environment and obesity, enhancing interagency coordination and partnerships, and examining evidence-based strategies for intervention. Results of this conference are now being considered in the planning of future research efforts.

Preventing and Treating Obesity Through Pharmacologic, Surgical, or Other Medical Approaches

Life-cycle of a fat cell:
A new series of NIH supported studies is characterizing how fat cells are formed and what determines their numbers and location in the body. Knowledge gained from this research will help in the understanding of obesity and other metabolic conditions.

Calcium as a potential supplement to prevent weight gain:
Intramural NIH investigators are studying the role of calcium supplementation for prevention of weight gain. An ongoing 340-person randomized, controlled clinical trial of dietary supplementation with 1500 mg/d of calcium carbonate will determine whether calcium intake, which is considered an easily modifiable dietary factor, can affect future weight gain in overweight and obese adults.

Investigations of drug therapy in children and adolescents:
Therapy for significantly overweight children and adolescents with obesity-related health conditions is also being studied by intramural investigators.

Two ongoing randomized, placebo-controlled trials in the NIH Intramural Research Program are studying promising pharmacologic interventions: metformin for children ages 6 to 12 years, and orlistat for adolescents, ages 12 to 17 years.

Bariatric surgery:
For people who are extremely obese, expected weight loss from behavior change alone may not be sufficient to have a major impact on health and is unlikely to be sustained. Bariatric surgical procedures, which restrict stomach size and/or lead to decreased absorption of nutrients, are being increasingly performed to treat severe obesity. These procedures can have dramatic benefits (such as improved glycemic control or even reversal of type 2 diabetes), but also carry substantial risks, including death. The NIH has now established a Bariatric Surgery Clinical Research Consortium, the Longitudinal Assessment of Bariatric Surgery (LABS), to facilitate and accelerate research in this area. This consortium will help pool the necessary clinical expertise and administrative resources to facilitate the conduct of multiple and novel clinical studies in a timely, efficient manner. Development of a database using standardized definitions, clinical protocols, and data collection instruments will enhance the ability to provide meaningful evidence-based recommendations for patient evaluation, selection, and follow-up care. This database, in turn, will promote rapid dissemination of research findings to healthcare professionals. In addition, this consortium will serve as a resource for basic and clinical studies which can explore the mechanisms by which surgery affects obesity-related comorbid conditions, energy expenditure, nutrient partitioning, appetitive behaviors, and psychosocial factors. This may lead to improved understanding of the factors underlying the development of obesity, with implications for new strategies for prevention and treatment.

Beyond BMI—Identifying additional traits associated with obesity that could facilitate large-scale genetics studies:
In rare cases, an individual may have a single genetic variation that leads to obesity, but for most obese people, the combined influences of variations in multiple genes likely contribute to excess weight gain. The search for genes that contribute to obesity may be greatly enhanced by the optimal selection of obesity-associated physical, molecular, or behavioral traits (phenotypes) to evaluate. Correlating the presence of an obesity-associated phenotype with a particular genetic variation can help lead scientists to genes that influence obesity. Although BMI, a measure of weight relative to height, has been useful for epidemiologic and other studies, other phenotypes may prove to be even more informative for genetic research. These may include, for example, traits measurable by imaging techniques, molecular analyses, and/or behavioral assessments. A recent NIH-sponsored workshop brought together external experts to recommend methods for measuring various obesity associated phenotypes that would be practical to implement in a large-scale human genetics study. As a result of this workshop, new initiatives are planned to take advantage of molecular tools in model organisms to

expand the list of potential drug targets and to link genetics to pre-obese metabolic states.

Longitudinal studies will be needed to connect genes, metabolism and subsequent development of obesity.

Enhancing research on mouse models by facilitating characterization of the mice:

The NIH has established a set of centers to provide, high quality metabolic and physiologic analysis of mouse models of obesity, diabetes, diabetic complications, and related disorders.

Source: National Institutes of Health (NIH).
Strategic Plan for NIH Obesity Research. NIH publication No. 04-5493.
Bethesda, MD: National Institutes of Health, 2004. Appendix B 69–75.

References

Bessesen, D. H. "Update on Obesity." *Journal of Clinical Endocrinology & Metabolism* 93, no. 6 (2008): 2027–2034.

Bish, C. L., H. M. Blanck, M. K. Serdula, M. Marcus, H. W. Kohl III, and L. K. Khan. "Diet and Physical Activity Behaviors among Americans Trying to Lose Weight: 2000 Behavioral Risk Factor Surveillance System." *Obesity Research* 13, no. 3 (2005): 596–607.

Burger King. "U.S. Nutritional Information: Core Menu Items January 2008." 2008. [Online information; retrieved 1/12/09.] http://www.bk.com/Nutrition/PDFs/brochure.pdf.

Centers for Disease Control and Prevention (CDC). "Childhood Overweight: Consequences." Atlanta: CDC, 2007.

Gardner, G., and B. Halweil. "Overfed and Underfed: The Global Epidemic of Malnutrition." Washington, DC: Worldwatch Institute, 2000.

Jack in the Box. "Burgers and More." 2008. [Online nutritional information; retrieved 1/12/09.] http://www.jackinthebox.com/ourfood/dynamic/nutrition.php?cat=1.

Jackson, A. S., and M. L. Pollock. "Generalized Equations for Predicting Body Density of Men." *British Journal of Nutrition* 40, no. 3 (1978): 497–504.

Jackson, A. S., M. L. Pollock, and A. Ward. "Generalized Equations for Predicting Body Density of Women." *Medicine & Science in Sports & Exercise* 12, no. 3 (1980): 175–181.

National Heart, Lung and Blood Institute (NHLBI). *Clinical Guidelines on the Identification, Evaluation, and Treatment of Overweight and Obesity in Adults: The Evidence Report.* Bethesda, MD: National Heart, Lung and Blood Institute, 1998.

National Heart, Lung and Blood Institute (NHLBI) and North American Association for the Studyof Obesity (NAASO). *The Practical Guide to the Identification, Evaluation, and Treatment of Overweight and Obesity in Adults.* NIH Publication Number 00-4084.Bethesda, MD: National Institutes of Health, 2000.

Ogden, C. L., M. D. Carroll, M. A. McDowell, and K. M. Flegal KM. "Obesity among Adults in the United States—No Change since 2003–2004." Hyattsville, MD: National Center for Health Statistics, 2007.

Putnam, J., J. Allshouse, and L. S. Kantor. "U.S. Per Capita Food Supply Trends: More Calories, Refined Carbohydrates, and Fats." *Food Review* 25, no. 3 (2002): 1–4.

Siri, W. E.. "Body Composition from Fluid Spaces and Density: Analysis of Methods. 1961." *Nutrition* 9, no. 5 (1993): 480–491; discussion 480, 492.

U.S. Department of Agriculture (USDA). "MyPyramid Food Intake Pattern Calorie Levels." 2005. [Online information; retrieved 1/12/09.] http://www.mypyramid.gov/downloads/MyPyramid_Calorie _Levels.pdf.

U.S. Department of Health and Human Services (HHS). "The Surgeon General's Call to Action to Prevent and Decrease Overweight and Obesity." Rockville, MD: Public Health Service, U.S. Department of Health and Human Services, 2001.

World Health Organization (WHO). "Obesity and Overweight." In *Global Strategy on Diet, Physical Activity and Health.* Geneva: WHO, 2008.

7

Directory of Agencies, Programs, and Organizations

S ome of the information provided below is adapted from the Web sites of the agencies, programs, and organizations listed below. Use common sense when accessing information, and ask the following questions: Does the organization have any special interest that might make them put a spin on the information? What is the source of funding? These questions should be considered when viewing all Web sites, including those that are consumer oriented as well as those from nonprofit organizations, industry, or the government.

The organizations are listed according to the following categories:

1. Government agents and national programs and initiatives
2. International agencies and organizations
3. Non-profit, professional, and trade organizations

Government Agencies and National Programs and Initiatives

National organizations have several functions. Some promote health (e.g., U.S. Department of Agriculture), study different diseases (e.g., National Institutes of Health), or collect and disseminate statistics about the health of the nation (e.g., Centers for Disease Control and Prevention).

Agricultural Research Service (ARS)
Jamie L. Whitten Building
1400 Independence Ave. SW
Washington, DC 20250
Phone: 202-720-3656
Web site: www.ars.usda.gov
E-mail: Agsec@usda.gov

ARS is the U.S. Department of Agriculture's (USDA) primary research agency for scientific information. Its research covers the study of agriculture anywhere from the growing fields to the dining table. ARS ensures that American agricultural products are safe and of good quality and competitive within the world economy. The agency also determines the best nutrition to keep people healthy throughout the life cycle. It has developed a number of high-fiber, low-calorie products that are used by food companies as fat substitutes. Oatrim, for example, is used in products such as frozen dinners and other products to lower their calorie and cholesterol content. The ARS National Research Program on Obesity aims to carry out research on obesity prevention by coordinating human nutrition with ARS crop studies, animal breeding, and new product and food-processing research. The agency's obesity research areas are based on learning what people eat, what the body needs, and how to modify foods to be more beneficial.

Center for Nutrition Policy and Promotion (CNPP)
3101 Park Center Drive, 10th Floor
Alexandria, VA 22302-1594
Phone: 703-305-7600
Fax: 703-305-3300
Web site: http://www.cnpp.usda.gov/

The Center for Nutrition Policy and Promotion, created in 1994, is an agency of the U.S. Department of Agriculture. It conducts research into consumer food behaviors in areas such as analysis in nutrition knowledge and attitudes, dietary survey methodology, and nutrition education techniques. Estimates of the overall nutrient content of the U.S. food supply, measured since 1909, are maintained by the CNPP. A staff of expert nutritionists, dietitians, economists, and policy experts link up-to-date scientific research with messages about healthful nutrition for the American public.

The Center is the agency that publishes and publicizes the *Dietary Guidelines for Americans*, which are the basis for government nutrition policy and nutrition education activities. The *Dietary Guidelines* are jointly reviewed and updated every five years by the USDA and the U.S. Department of Health and Human Services (HHS). The CNPP develops educational tools to help Americans put the *Dietary Guidelines* into practice such as the Food Guide Pyramid, MyPyramid Tracker, MyPyramid for Kids, Steps to a Healthier Weight, and, more recently, MyPyramid PodCasts.

Centers for Disease Control and Prevention (CDC)
1600 Clifton Road
Atlanta, GA 30333
Phone: 404-498-1515, 800-311-3435
Web site:http://www.cdc.gov
E-mail: cdcinfo@cdc.gov

CDC, under the Department of Health and Human Services, is the agency that tracks and investigates public health trends. It publishes weekly data on all deaths and diseases reported in the United States in the publication *Morbidity and Mortality Weekly Report*.The Web site is a frequently updated resource for fact sheets related to obesity prevention and provides an interactive body mass index calculator.

CDC created the Division of Nutrition, Physical Activity and Obesity (DNPAO) to help prevent and control obesity by promoting regular physical activity and good nutrition. The Division's obesity prevention activities include translating results of research into practical advice for medical professionals and the public. The Research to Practice Series discusses the implications of the newest studies on nutrition, physical activity, and obesity research. The series includes free tools, such as print-ready brochures and PowerPoint programs, for health professionals to summarize and translate scientific evidence for the general public. Some series offerings are "How to Use Fruits and Vegetables to Help Manage Your Weight" and "Do Increased Portion Sizes Affect How Much We Eat?" Another DNPAO activity is promoting obesity prevention and control at work sites. The Division conducts demonstration projects at CDC work sites and then adapts effective strategies into interactive Web-based tools that employers cans use to design their own programs. Physical activity guidelines are also being developed in partnership with the President's Council on Physical Fitness and Sports. On an international basis, DNPAO collaborates with the World Health Organization as leaders in building worldwide research to study effective public health practices that may combat obesity.

Economic Research Service (ERS)
1800 M Street NW
Washington, DC 20036-5831
Phone: 1-800-999-6779
Web site:http://www.ers.usda.gov/
E-mail: InfoCenter@ers.usda.gov

ERS is part of the U.S. Department of Agriculture. Its job is to be the primary source of economic information and research about food and farming for policy makers and the public. One of five areas of ERS research is a goal to promote a healthy, well-nourished population. With respect to obesity, data are used to study how obesity is affected by food supply and national eating patterns. ERS publishes consumer-friendly reports and *Amber Waves*, a magazine that contains in-depth feature articles, research findings, and previews of ongoing research.

Food and Drug Administration (FDA)
5600 Fishers Lane
Rockville, MD 20857-0001
Phone: 1-888-463-6332
Web site: http://www.fda.gov
Contact: http://www.fda.gov/comments.html

The FDA is a federal regulatory agency within HHS. It reviews toxicological research and clinical trials in order to approve or reject new drugs for the marketplace. The FDA Center for Food Safety and Applied Nutrition is responsible for taking action against any unsafe dietary supplement after it reaches the market. The FDA relies on consumers reports of serious events through the MedWatch Program. An example of FDA action against unsafe dietary supplements was the case of ephedrine-containing weight-loss products. Numerous adverse events were reported to the administration, including chest pain, heart attacks, strokes, and death. In 2004, the FDA issued a ruling prohibiting the sales of dietary supplements containing ephedrine.

The FDA Web site has useful information for consumers and educators. Topics include dietary supplements, food labeling and nutrition, medical devices, and drugs. A free electronic newsletter about dietary supplements often contains information about ingredients used in weight-loss products. The site also provides information about the FDA program to combat obesity.

Food and Nutrition Service (FNS)
3101 Park Center Drive
Alexandria, VA 22302
Phone: 703-305-2281
Web site and contact: http://www.fns.usda.gov/fns/
default.htm

The Food and Nutrition Service is a branch of the USDA that serves to provide families and children in need with easier access to nutritious foods through education and food assistance programs. FNS is responsible for the National School Lunch Program; Food Stamp Program; and Women, Infant and Children Food Assistance Program. FNS recognizes that obesity is a serious health concern in the United States, and its goal is to educate the public, especially children in school, so that they can make healthy food choices.

HealthierUS
U.S. Department of Health and Human Services
Office of Public Health and Science
Office of Disease Prevention and Health Promotion
1101 Wootton Parkway, Suite LL100
Rockville, MD 20852
Phone: 240-453-8280
Web site: www.healthierUS.gov
E-mail: info@nhic.org

The HealthierUS initiative was started by President George W. Bush in 2002. The underlying premise is that increasing personal fitness and becoming healthier are critical steps to achieving a better and longer life. The initiative focuses on promotion of four key messages: (1) be physically active every day, (2) eat a nutritious diet, (3) get preventive screenings, and (4) make healthy choices.

At the level of the federal government, the President's Council on Physical Fitness and Sports was revitalized, and certain federal agencies were directed to review their policies related to the four areas and propose revisions, including new actions.

Media-Smart Youth: Eat, Think, and Be Active
P.O. Box 3006
Rockville, MD 20847
Phone: 800-370-2943
Web site: http://www.nichd.nih.gov/msy/
E-mail: NICHDInformationResourceCenter@mail.nih.gov

Created by the Eunice Kennedy Shriver National Institute of Child Health and Human Development, Media-Smart Youth is an after-school program designed to educate young people ages 11 to 13 on how the media can lead to poor health choices in their lives. Educating children about the media is important because many children spend hours watching television, playing video games, or surfing the Web. All of these activities take time away from physical activity. This is not specifically an obesity prevention program, but it helps young people to think critically about how media have a major influence on their attitudes about health so they can make smart choices about nutrition and physical activity. This program is available to after-school providers or activity leaders to help encourage children to be active every day.

National Cancer Institute (NCI)
NCI Public Inquiries Office
6116 Executive Boulevard
Room 3036A
Bethesda, MD 20892-8322
Phone: 800-422-6237
Web site: www.cancer.gov
E-mail: cancergovstaff@mail.nih.gov.

NCI was established in 1937 under the National Cancer Institute Act and is part of the National Institutes of Health (NIH). NCI is involved with research, education, training, and support for cancer centers. NCI has funded several studies relating obesity and cancer risks. Its Web site provides fact sheets that make the research studies understandable to the general public.

National Heart, Lung and Blood Institute (NHLBI)
P.O. Box 30105
Bethesda, MD 20824-0105
Phone: 301-592-8573
Web site: http://www.nhlbi.nih.gov/index.htm
E-mail: nhlbiinfo@nhlbi.nih.gov

NHLBI is part of NIH. Its primary mission is to support basic and applied research related to heart, lung, and blood diseases. NHLBI established the Obesity Education Initiative (OEI) in 1991 to help decrease the incidence of cardiovascular disease and type 2 diabetes by reducing the prevalence of overweight and increasing physical activity in Americans. The OEI uses both population-based and high-risk-individual strategies to further its goals. The population approach focuses on the general population with activities that include promotion of physical education and a nutrition curriculum in schools nationwide and Hearts N' Parks, a community-based venture in partnership with the National Recreation and Park Association, to encourage increased physical activity every day. The high-risk category of tactics targets individuals who are experiencing, or are at increased risk for, the adverse health effects associated with overweight and obesity. To provide a basis for intervention, an expert panel issued the *Clinical Guidelines on the Identification, Evaluation, and Treatment of Overweight and Obesity in Adults: The Evidence Report* in June 1998. It enumerated the first federal clinical practice guidelines that analyze overweight and obesity issues using an evidence-based approach and provided practical strategies for applying the recommendations.

NHLBI offers education activities for health care professionals and holds conferences for researchers at the NIH center. The Web site offers a wealth of information for the public, health professionals, and researchers. The site includes the latest health news, tools, and tutorials. Online slides and an electronic textbook on obesity also can be viewed. NHLBI provides patient and public obesity treatment recommendations in its *Aim for a Healthy Weight* guide.

National Institute of Diabetes and Digestive and Kidney Diseases (NIDDK)
Office of Communications & Public Liaison
Building 31, Room 9A06
31 Center Drive, MSC 2560
Bethesda, MD 20892-2560
Phone: 301-496-3583
Web site: http://www.niddk.nih.gov

NIDDK is one of the institutes at NIH. It conducts and supports basic and clinical research on diabetes and digestive and kidney diseases. Within NIDDK is the Office of Obesity Research; this office is part of NIDDK because obesity is estimated to be a precipitating cause for 80 percent of type 2 diabetes and its complications. Given that obesity and its medical costs are increasing, and to emphasize the importance of obesity, some researchers suggest that NIDDK's name should be changed to National Institute of Obesity, Diabetes, and Digestive and Kidney Diseases (NIODDK).

The NIDDK Web site has a section titled Health Information for the Public. Weight control is one of the topics (see also the entry on Weight-control Information Network below).

National Institutes of Health (NIH)
9000 Rockville Pike
Bethesda, MD 20892
Phone: 301-496-4000
Web site: http://www.nih.gov/about/contact.htm (includes addresses for the 27 institutes and centers)
E-mail: NIHinfo@od.nih.gov

The National Institutes of Health is part of HHS. It is the chief federal agency responsible for conducting and supporting research. NIH obesity studies range from small pilot projects to multicenter clinical trials and include lifestyle, pharmacological, and other approaches. The research focuses on diagnosis, prevention, and treatment as well as building a scientific evidence base for public policy decisions. A major NIH objective is to develop ways to explain research results from clinical trials to the medical community and the public. NIH is appropriated about $28 billion annually by the U.S. Congress. Eighty percent of this money is used for funding research grants in the United States and some foreign countries.

In 2004, the NIH Obesity Research Task Force published the *Strategic Plan for NIH Obesity Research*, a multifaceted agenda for the study of behavioral and environmental causes of obesity in conjunction with the study of genetic and biologic causes. The plan detailed coordination of obesity research across NIH.

The names of the 27 institutes and centers reflect their emphasis, such as National Heart, Lung and Blood Institute, National Cancer Institute, National Institute of Allergy and Infectious Diseases, National Institute on Alcohol Abuse and Alcoholism, and Center for Complementary and Alternative Medicine. There is not a National Institute of Obesity, despite obesity's economic and health impacts on American people.

National Recreation and Park Association (NRPA)
22377 Belmont Ridge Road
Ashburn, VA 20148
Phone: 703- 858-2162
Fax: 703-729-4753
Web site: http://www.nrpa.org
E-mail: info@nrpa.org

NRPA has expertise in mobilizing communities, providing community-based physical activity programs, and identifying barriers to physical activity. The agency formed a partnership with NHLBI to get Americans moving to help reduce overweight and obesity.

Office of the Surgeon General (OSG)
5600 Fishers Lane, Room 18-66
Rockville, MD 20857
Phone: 301-443-4000
Web site: www.surgeongeneral.gov/topics/obesity
Contact: http://www.surgeongeneral.gov/contactus.html

The OSG is part of the Department of Health and Human Services. The surgeon general, appointed by the president, is a commissioned officer in the Public Health Service who holds the rank of a three-star vice admiral while in office.

One of the jobs of the surgeon general is to provide the best scientific information about how to improve health and reduce the risk of illness and injury. Its Childhood Overweight and Obesity Prevention initiative includes sections titled "Overweight and Obesity: Health Consequences" and "Overweight and Obesity: What You Can Do." Its Web site contains the report "The Surgeon General's Call to Action to Prevent and Decrease Overweight and Obesity," in addition to information on health consequences of obesity.

U.S. Department of Agriculture (USDA)
1400 Independence Ave. SW
Washington, DC 20250
Web site: http://www.usda.gov
E-mail for secretary of Agriculture: AgSec@usda.gov

The USDA is the primary government agency for agriculture, food, and human nutrition. It has a number of divisions, including the Agricultural Research Service and Economic Research Service. One of its mission areas is to improve health in the United States. For example, the USDA's Center for Nutrition Policy and Promotion links scientific research to dietary guidance, nutrition policy coordination, and nutrition education. The Web site provides a link to the *Dietary Guidelines for Americans* as well as information about physical activity and long-term weight loss. The USDA's National Agricultural Library is accessible by e-mail (http://www.nal.usda.gov) where requests can be made for copies of published research articles. Navigating this site is difficult in part because of the many links. However, it is worth the time to explore because of the extensive amount of information about obesity available there.

U.S. Department of Health and Human Services (HHS)
200 Independence Ave. SW
Washington, DC 20201
Phone: 202-619-0257, 1-877-696-6775
Web site: http://www.hhs.gov
Contact: http://www.hhs.gov/feedback.html

HHS is the United States' primary government agency that aims to protect the health of Americans. It has 11 operating divisions to administer more than 300 programs. Some of these divisions include NIH, FDA, and CDC. The 2005 *Dietary Guidelines for Americans* and "The Surgeon General's Call to Action" releases are published by HHS. Its Web site features daily health tips, which are available in audio and text format, and links to other sites, such as Healthier US.gov, which provides information on physical fitness, nutrition, and how to make healthy choices. Interactive games are also available to help children and teens learn about healthy eating and physical fitness.

Weight-control Information Network (WIN)
National Institute of Diabetes and Digestive and Kidney Disease
1 WIN Way
Bethesda, MD 20892-3665
Phone: 877- 946-4627
Web site: http://www.win.niddk.nih.gov/
E-mail: win@info.niddk.nih.gov

WIN is an information service of the NIDDK at the National Institutes of Health. Its focus is on getting up-to-date, science-based information to the public and media about weight control. WIN's information covers the range from underweight to normal weight to obesity. WIN provides information about risks associated with overweight/obesity, with special emphasis on diabetes. Its booklets, some of which can be downloaded through its Web site, cover topics such as determining a healthy weight, being active no matter one's size, bariatric surgery, and treating obesity using prescription medications. Many of the booklets are also in Spanish. WIN encourages anyone to duplicate and distribute copies of any of the booklets, as the information on the WIN Web site is not copyrighted.

International Agencies and Organizations

Food and Agricultural Organization of the United Nations (FAO)
Liaison Office
2175 K Street NW, Suite 500
Washington, DC 20037
Phone: 202-653-2400
Web site: http://fao.org
E-mail for world headquarters: FAO-HQ@fao.org

FAO is one of the agencies of the United Nations. Its major activity in the area of food and nutrition is an international effort to reduce malnutrition and hunger. Although obesity is not as big a problem as is hunger, it is rapidly increasing in developing nations. FAO identifies the problem in the report *The Nutrition Transition and Obesity.* FAO's approach to preventing the problem from getting worse is to educate the public in every country. FAO's objectives are to promote good nutrition and physical activity and agriculture policy that encourage the consumption of healthy foods.

Health Canada (HC)
Public Affairs
BrookeClaxton Building
Ottawa, Ontario K1A 0K9
Canada
Web site: http://www.hc-sc.gc.ca/index-eng.php
E-mail: Info@hc-sc.gc.ca

Health Canada is the national department responsible for helping Canadians achieve good health while respecting individual choices and circumstances. The HC Office of Nutrition Policy and Promotion defines, promotes, and implements evidence-based nutrition policies and standards.

The Web site provides information about health-related legislation and activities and has a page called Healthy Living, where articles can be retrieved such as "Obesity (Its Your Health)," "Risk Factors for Heart Disease," and "Canada's Food Guide to Healthy Eating." It also provides links to other Canadian government sites that contain additional information about obesity.

International Association for the Study of Obesity (IASO)
231 North Gower Street
London NW1 2NR
United Kingdom
Phone: +44-0-20 7691 1900
Web site: www.iaso.org
E-mail: enquiries@iaso.org

IASO is a registered charity in the United Kingdom. It is an international organization that serves as an umbrella for 52 national obesity associations representing 56 countries. As a representative organization, it works for development of effective policies for obesity prevention and management throughout the world. Its Web site features an obesity experts forum as well as links to journals specializing in research on obesity and related health problems. IASO publishes the *International Journal of Obesity*, the *International Journal of Pediatric Obesity*, and *Obesity Reviews*. Another Web site features is "Latest News," which provides links to relevant activities and meetings of organizations that are doing obesity research.

International Federation for the Surgery of Obesity (IFSO)
IFSO Executive Secretariat
Bruennsteinstr. 10
81541 Munich
Germany
Phone: +49-89-4141 92 50
Fax: +49-89-4141 92 45
Web site: www.isfo.com
E-mail: Heather.Wynn@medc.de

IFSO is an innternational organization that serves as an umbrella for 34 national associations of bariatric surgeons. Its goal is to bring together surgeons and allied health professionals such as anesthesiologists, dietitians, internists, nurse practitioners, nutritionists, and psychologists who are involved in the treatment of very obese patients. The main goal of IFSO is to optimize the treatment of severely obese patients. The organization has also produced a set of guidelines for selection criteria for patients and minimal requirements for bariatric surgeons. IFSO is committed to creating a system of accreditation for individual surgeons and bariatric centers around the world. The Web site contains information about treatments, scientific articles, and meetings. IFSO organizes a yearly World Congress, which, along with its online forum, provides an opportunity for surgeons to exchange knowledge on surgical treatment of severely obese patients; to present new techniques, research, and concepts; and to meet the experts in the field. The Web site also has interactive movies about obesity discussing causes and risks as well as descriptions of various bariatric surgical procedures. It provides links to its publication *Obesity Surgery Journal* as well as a listing of bariatric surgeons.

International Obesity Taskforce (IOTF)
231 North Gower Street
London NW1 2NR
United Kingdom
Phone: +44-0-20 7691 1900
Web site: www.iotf.org
E-mail: inquiries@iaso.org / obesity@iotf.org

IOTF is part of the International Association for the Study of Obesity. It works with partners in the Global Prevention Alliance to support new strategies to improve diet and activity and prevent obesity. As a global network of experts on obesity and the advocacy arm of IASO, IOTF works with the World Health Organization and other private and public groups. With a special emphasis on preventing childhood obesity, its goal is to alert people around the world about the urgency of the obesity problem and to persuade governments to act now. Publications and research news about a range of obesity-related issues can be accessed through the IOTF Web site. The site also presents useful links to government agencies, academic institutions, and resources for health-related information.

World Health Organization (WHO)
United Nations Liaison Office
1889 F Street, NW, Room 369
Washington, DC 20006
Phone: 202-974-3299
Web site: http://www.who.int/en/
E-mail: info@who.int.

WHO is the directing and coordinating authority for health within the United Nations. It has six general goals, including promoting development; fostering health security; strengthening health systems; harnessing research, information, and evidence; improving performance; and enhancing partnerships. In 2002, WHO worked with FAO to issue the joint Expert Consultation *Diet, Nutrition and the Prevention of Chronic Diseases*. This publication was followed in May 2004 by WHO's landmark Global Strategy on Diet, Physical Activity and Health (DPAS), developed to promote healthy lifestyles for adults and children in all countries. DPAS is a framework to reduce noncommunicable diseases such as obesity, diabetes, and cardiovascular disease by modifying risk factors of unhealthy diet and physical inactivity. In the area of obesity, WHO partners with the International Association for the Study of Obesity, primarily through the International Obesity Taskforce. The WHO Web site provides a wealth of fascinating information about international health topics, programs and projects, and interactive pages with data and statistics about obesity in individual countries around the world.

Nonprofit, Professional, and Trade Organizations

American Academy of Family Physicians (AAFP)
1140 Tomahawk Creek Parkway
Leawood, KS 66211
Phone: 800-274-2237
Web site: www.aafp.org

AAFP, a national organization, represents 94,000 family physicians, family medicine residents, and medical students. The organization has released a guide for family physicians to help their overweight patients and launched a 10-year fitness initiative called Americans in Motion. The organization asserts that ample evidence supports recognizing both childhood overweight and adult obesity as diseases and reimbursement from insurance companies to family physicians who provide reasonable diagnosis and treatment of overweight and obesity. The Web site has a number of sections that provide excellent information for families, including answers to common questions and weight issues for children. Links to other sites are available as well (e.g., HHS, Office of Disease Prevention and Health Promotion, Reuters Health), which provide information about obesity. AAFP produces a semi-monthly, peer-reviewed journal entitled *American Family Physician.*

American Academy of Pediatrics (AAP)
141 Northwest Point Blvd.
Elk Grove Village, IL 60007-1098
Phone: 847-434-4000
Fax: 847-434-8000
Web site: www.aap.org/obesity
E-mail: kidsdocs@aap.org

AAP is a national professional association for pediatricians dedicated to the health of all infants, children, adolescents, and young adults. AAP was instrumental in developing a major breakthrough in medical policies and guidelines for childhood obesity as part of the important publication "Expert Committee Recommendations Regarding the Prevention, Assessment, and, Treatment of Child and Adolescents." The AAP Web site has links to tools and books for patients and parents including Parenting Corner Q&A and *A Parent's Guide to Childhood Obesity: A Road Map to Health*, which offers practical advice on how parents can help their children manage their weight. The site also has information about high blood pressure and children and cautions about the increased risk in children who are overweight. *Pediatrics*, the peer-reviewed journal of the AAP, has been published since January 1948.

American Cancer Society (ACS)
P.O. Box22538
Oklahoma City, OK 73123-1538
Phone: 866-228-4327
Web site: www.cancer.org
Contact: http://www.cancer.org/asp/contactUs/cus
_global.asp

ACS is a nonprofit organization funded by donations. It is dedicated to helping patients and their friends and family learn more about cancer. The ACS Web site is extensive and informative. People can get help in making decisions about cancer treatment and finding treatment centers. A survivor network is also coordinated through ACS's Web site. ACS's advocacy activities have influenced Congress and state governments and the organization has been instrumental in obtaining more than $1 billion annually for the National Cancer Institute for research.

With respect to obesity, people who are overweight or obese are at increased risk for developing certain cancers, and ACS presents research about the relationship between obesity and cancer. A page entitled "Take Control of Your Weight" includes guidelines for weight loss and a chance to plan a healthful diet with a virtual dietitian. Many of the materials on the site have been translated into Spanish and several Asian languages.

American College of Physicians (ACP)
190 North Independence Mail West
Philadelphia, PA 19106-1572
Phone: 800-523-1546
Web site: http://acponline.org/
Contact: http://www.acponline.org/cgi-bin/feedback

ACP is a national organization of physicians who specialize in the prevention, detection, and treatment of chronic illnesses such as diabetes and obesity. Established in 1915, ACP is a membership organization for physicians who treat adults. It publishes the *Annals of Internal Medicine*, a widely cited medical journal. On its Web site is a section for patients with information about obesity. The Internal Medicine Report section gives access to published papers and videos about important medical and health issues.

American College of Preventive Medicine (ACPM)
1307 New York Ave., N.W., Suite 200
Washington, DC 20005
Phone: 202-466-2044
Fax: 202-466-2662
Web site: www.acpm.org
E-mail: info@acpm.org

ACPM is a national professional society for U.S. doctors. The organization of about 2,000 members focuses on disease prevention and health promotion in individuals and in population groups. Preventive medicine–trained physicians work in primary care, in public health and government agencies, in workplaces, and in academia. ACPM has released an official position statement about the optimal diet for weight control that discourages the use of fad diets. The organization sponsors the *American Journal of Preventive Medicine* and a series of articles, some of which are related to obesity. However, these articles are only available to members and thus the direct impact on the public is limited.

American College of Sports Medicine (ACSM)
401 West Michigan Street
Indianapolis, IN 46202-3233
Phone 317-637-9200

Web site: http://acsm.org
Contact: http://www.acsm.org/_frm/departments/
indexnew.asp?area=general

ACSM is a nonprofit organization whose 20,000 members have expertise in the areas of sports medicine, exercise physiology, physical activity, and cardiovascular health. ACSM collaborates with other organizations and issues consensus statements. These so-called Position Stands are published in the College's scientific journal, *Medicine & Science in Sports & Exercise*. The ACSM Web site has a news release section that provides information about obesity and nutrition, including "Dispelling the Top 10 Nutrition Myths."

American Council on Science and Health (ACSH)
1995 Broadway, 2nd Floor
New York, NY 10023-5860
Phone: 866-905-2694
Fax: 212-362-4919
Web site: http://acsh.org
E-mail: acsh@acsh.org

ACSH is a nonprofit, consumer education consortium. Its board of experts comprises 350 physicians, scientists, and policy advisers. These experts review ACSH reports and participate in educational activities. ACSH is concerned with issues relating to food, nutrition, chemicals, pharmaceuticals, lifestyle, the environment, and health. Some of its publications include "Health Effects of Obesity," "Foods are not Cigarettes: Why Tobacco Lawsuits Are Not a Model for Obesity Lawsuits," and "Childhood Obesity." The News Center section of its Web site displays a list of articles from ACSH that have been published in the popular press. ACSH receives much of its funding from industry.

American Diabetes Association (ADiabA)
1701 North Beauregard Street
Alexandria, VA 22311
Phone: 1-800-342-2383
Web site: www.diabetes.org
E-mail: stepoutadmin@diabetes.org

The American Diabetes Association is a nonprofit health organization whose mission is to find ways to prevent, cure, and manage diabetes. It funds research, publishes scientific findings, and provides information and other services to people with diabetes. Both consumers and health professionals may become members. Because the American Diabetes Association and the American Dietetic Association are both referred to as ADA, for our purposes we refer to the American Diabetes Association as ADiabA and to the American Dietetic Association as ADietA. There is excellent information about obesity on the ADiabA Web site. For example, it has sections on weight loss and exercise, recipes for healthy eating, research updates, and an easy-to-use body mass index calculator.

American Dietetic Association (ADietA)
120 South Riverside Plaza, Suite 2000
Chicago, IL 60606
Phone: 800-877-1600
Web site: www.eatright.org
E-mail: media@eatright.org

ADietA, in contrast to ADiabA, is a professional organization of dietitians with expertise in nutrition, food, and health. ADietA is the largest organization of food and nutrition professionals in the world, with more than 68,000 members. Dietitians play an important role in helping people manage and prevent overweight and obesity by showing them how to formulate reasonable weight goals and personalized eating patterns that can be sustained over the long term. ADietA publishes the *Journal of the American Dietetic Association* and position papers on health issues, including weight control. The Web site has a variety of information about food and nutrition as well as a referral service that can link consumers with registered dietetic professionals. It also provides daily nutrition news and interesting tidbits of information. For example, in the United States, the average amount of weight that a new college student gains is about 15 pounds; this phenomenon is called the "freshman 15." In Canada, new students' weight gain is only 5 pounds and is known as the "freshman 5."

American Heart Association (AHA)
National Center
7272 Greenville Avenue
Dallas, TX 75231
Phone: 1-800-242-8721
Web site: www.americanheart.org
Contact: http://www.americanheart.org/presenter.jhtml?
identifier=10000046&title=generalquestions

AHA is a nonprofit, national voluntary health agency with professional and public members. The organization supports heart disease research, scientific meetings, and advocacy. It publishes several scientific journals and magazines for people concerned about prevention and treatment of heart disease. A subscription to *Heart Insight*, a quarterly patient magazine, is free to people who live in the United States. On the Web site, at HeartHub, there is a video on healthy eating, a body mass index calculator, and tips on eating well and losing weight. Downloadable publications are available in both English and Spanish, such as "How Can I Manage My Weight?" (*¿Cómo puedo controlar mi peso?*), and "Losing Weight the Healthy Way" (*Controlando su peso*).

American Institute for Cancer Research (AICR)
1759 R Street NW
Washington, DC 20009
Phone: 1-800-843-8114
Web site: www.aicr.org
E-mail: aicrweb@aicr.org

AICR encourages research on the relationship of nutrition, physical activity, and weight management to cancer risk; interprets the scientific literature; and educates the public about the results.

It also supports health professionals with educational materials and advice in planning programs on diet, nutrition, and cancer prevention. AICR's second expert report, *Nutrition, Physical Activity, and the Prevention of Cancer: A Global Perspective*, confirmed the relationship between excess body fat and increased cancer risk. AICR experts stressed that many cancers are preventable. In fact, maintaining a healthy weight may be the single most important way to protect against cancer.

Information on its Web site changes often in response to popular news stories. The section Ever Green, Ever Hungry featured articles about preventing winter weight gain and findings linking food, activity, and body weight to risk of colon cancer. One article listed is "Eat to Satisfy your Body—Not to Satisfy Your Friends." Subscription to AICR's e-newsletter is free.

American Medical Association (AMA)
515 N. State Street
Chicago, IL 60610
Phone: 800-621-8335
Web site: www.ama-assn.org

AMA, founded in 1847, is a membership organization of physicians. It publishes one of the most widely read medical journals, the *Journal of the American Medical Association*. In collaboration with the U.S. Department of Health and Human Services and the Robert Wood Johnson Foundation, AMA has published a series of clinical guidelines entitled Roadmaps for Clinical Practice. *Case Studies in Disease Prevention and Health Promotion*, one of the publications in this series, contains booklets that provide specific, focused tactics to identify and treat diseases such as obesity during routine medical care. The "Assessment and Management of Adult Obesity" road map is available online (AMA 2007). In January 2007, AMA released the report *Expert Committee Recommendations on the Assessment, Prevention, and Treatment of Child and Adolescent Overweight and Obesity*, which will have far-reaching effects on how childhood obesity is identified and treated in the United States. The AMA Web site provides links to reports, publications, and resources about the health effects of overweight and obesity.

American Public Health Association (APHA)
800 I Street NW
Washington, DC 20001-3710
Phone: 202-777-2742 (APHA)
Web site: www.apha.org
E-mail: comments@apha.org

APHA is a public health organization that has been working to improve public health since 1872. The Association's goal is to protect Americans from preventable health threats and to ensure that health promotion, disease prevention, and preventive health services are accessible to everyone in the United States. As an organization, it works with members of Congress, regulatory agencies, and other public health organizations to influence policies and set priorities on a wide variety of issues that include children's health, managed care, disease control, health disparities, bioterrorism, international health, and tobacco control. The APHA has announced that preventing obesity in children is one of the most important public health issues facing the United States today. It encourages development of new approaches and partnerships to address the problem. The Association issues policy statements about obesity prevention, including "Support for Nutrition Labeling in Fast-Food and Other Chain Restaurants" in 2005 and "Urgent Call for a Nationwide Public Health Infrastructure and Action to Reverse the Obesity Epidemic" in 2006. In the *American Journal of Public Health*, published for public health workers and academics, special emphasis is given to analysis of current public health issues in a historical context.

The Web site provides tools and plans for both individual and community efforts to tackle obesity. Its newsroom has topical press releases such as "Purchasing Behavior Influenced by Calorie Information. It Worked for Jared!" (see the biographical profiles of Jared Fogle in Chapter 5). This topic of this press release, a study of New York City fast-food chains, demonstrated that when calorie information was displayed on deli cases near the register, consumers bought food containing about 52 fewer calories.

American Society of Bariatric Physicians (ASBM)
2821 South Parker Road, Suite 625
Aurora, CO 80014
Phone: 303-770-2526
Web site: http://www.asbp.org/
E-mail: jrobinson@nasbp.org

ASBM is a national medical society of doctors offering medical treatment of obesity (bariatrics), weight loss, and dieting. Its Web site has a section for the public (Frequently Asked Questions) about the growing problem of obesity and tips on weight loss. The Locate a Physician section lists names, addresses, and phone numbers of bariatric physicians. Currently no evaluation mechanism is in place to regulate the quality of physicians.

ASBM's Web site contains up-to-date information and news about the field of obesity treatment and medical weight loss.

American Society for Metabolic and Bariatric
Surgery (ASMBS)
100 SW 75th Street, Suite 201
Gainesville, FL 32607
Phone: 352-331-4900
Web site: www.asbs.org
E-mail: info@asmbs.org

ASMBM was founded in 1983. It is a nonprofit medical organization made up of surgeons and other healthcare professionals. As declared on the home page of its Web site, its vision "is to improve public health and well being by lessening the burden of the disease of obesity and related diseases throughout the world." It publishes the scientific journal *Surgery for Obesity and Related Diseases*. ASMBS offers educational programs for physicians, other health care professionals, and the public about bariatric surgery and guidelines for ethical patient selection and care. The Society promotes outcome studies and measures of quality assurance to improve the safety and effectiveness of obesity surgeries.

The Web site has accessible information about extreme obesity, bariatric surgery, and diabetes. A section helps calculate BMI and assigns an obesity classification based on BMI. For example, Class I Obesity is a BMI ranging from 30 to 34.9.

Calorie Control Council (CCC)
5775 Peachtree-Dunwoody Road, Suite 500-G
Atlanta, GA 30342
Phone: 404-252-3663
Web site: http://www.caloriecontrol.org/
E-mail: webmaster@caloriecontrol.org

The Calorie Control Council is nonprofit organization supported by 60 companies that manufacture or sell low-calorie and reduced-fat foods and beverages. The Council provides understandable information about low-calorie sweeteners like aspartame, saccharin, and sucralose and about fat replacers like polydextrose and olestra for consumers interested cutting dietary calories and fat. CCC has sponsored research on low-calorie ingredients, foods, and beverages including studies about safety, metabolism, consumer use, and public opinion of food additives.

Center for Consumer Freedom (CCF)
P.O. Box 34557
Washington, DC 20043
Phone: 202-463-7112
Web site: http://www.consumerfreedom.com
E-mail: http://www.consumerfreedom.com/contact.cfm

CCF is a nonprofit organization whose mission is to promote personal responsibility and protect consumer choice through activism and print, radio, and television advertisements like the one entitled "You Are Too Stupid ... to make your own food choices." Each year, CCF issues its Tarnished Halo awards to animal-rights and environmental activists, public interest advocates, trial lawyers, and food and beverage crusaders who claim that they know what is best for the general public. CCF has opposed the regulation of the food and restaurant industry. For example, it is against posting calories on menu boards of fast-food restaurant chains.

Center for Science in the Public Interest (CSPI)
1875 Connecticut Ave. NW, Suite 300
Washington, DC 20009
Phone: 202-332-9110
Web site: www.cspinet.org

Founded in 1971, CSPI is an advocacy organization for science-based information about nutrition and health, food safety, alcohol policy, and sound science. CSPI's goals are to counter the food industry's influence on public opinion and public policies and to lobby for government policies that are consistent with scientific evidence. CSPI also aims to educate the public. Its monthly newsletter, *Nutrition Action Health letter*, has about 900,000 subscribers in the United States and Canada. It periodically reviews fad diets and issues about overweight and obesity. CSPI has been on the forefront of the efforts to require nutrition facts on packaged foods and to have calories of fast foods available at the point of purchase. It has also conducted studies on the nutrition quality of restaurant meals. CSPI works to improve food safety in an effort to decrease the number of food-borne illnesses. Its Web site has a section devoted to obesity. The section Current Press Releases has displayed such items as "New Poll Shows Calories Hard for New Yorkers to Guess" and "With Calories Hard to Guess, Washington Voters Want Answers on Menus."

Consumers Union (CU)
1101 17th Street, NW, Suite 500
Washington, DC 20036
Phone: 202-462-6262
Fax: 202-265-6262
Web site: http://consumersunion.org
Contact: http://custhelp.consumerreports.org/cgi-bin/consumerreports.cfg/php/enduser/ask.php

CU is a nonprofit, independent testing and information organization. It publishes *Consumer Reports*. It does not accept advertisements so as to remain independent of bias. CU has reviewed weight-loss supplements and diets and diet programs. Because many consumers log on to the Web for weight-loss advice, *Consumer Reports* has rated dieting information sites and ranked the ones that are most helpful. The *Consumer Reports* Web site features a page entitled "4 Ways to Keep Your Child at a Healthy Weight."

Council on Size and Weight Discrimination (CSWD)
P.O. Box 305
Mt. Marion, NY 12456
Phone: 610-70-8166
Web site: http://cswd.org
E-mail: info@cswd.org

CSWD is a nonprofit group that is working to change attitudes about body weight on the job, in the media, and for medical treatment. Its Web site has pages with facts and suggestions such as "How to Fight Weight Discrimination," "10 Steps to Loving Your Body Just As It Is," and "Ten Reasons to Give Up Dieting." It also presents information and guidelines on how to become active in fighting weight discrimination.

Endocrine Society
8401 Connecticut Avenue, Suite 900
Chevy Chase, MD 20815
Phone: 301-941-0200
Web site: http://www.endo-society.org
E-mail: societyservices@endo-society.org

The Endocrine Society, formed in 1916, supports research on hormones and the clinical practice of endocrinology. Worldwide, it has more than 14,000 members who represent medicine, molecular and cellular biology, genetics, immunology, education, industry, and health care fields. The members are committed to research and treatment of endocrine disorders, including diabetes, infertility, osteoporosis, thyroid disease, and obesity and lipid abnormalities.

The Society has developed clinical practice guidelines that are offered to clinicians as the most recent advances and new strategies to improve care by reducing variations in practice, reducing medical errors, and providing consistent quality of care for diagnosing and treating obese or overweight patients. The Society selects topics for guidelines by examining areas where no guidelines are in place or where existing guidelines are out-of-date. Each guideline is created by a task force of experts who rely on evidence-based reviews of the literature to provide support for the recommendations. In 2007, the Endocrine Society released the guideline "Prevention and Treatment of Pediatric Obesity." The guideline's recommendations include defining childhood overweight and obesity using BMI percentiles and supporting diet and physical activity modification as the cornerstones of prevention and as a prerequisite for other treatment. The group advocates that schools encourage and allow 60 minutes of moderate to vigorous daily exercise in all grades. The guideline also discusses policies for bariatric surgery in young people. The Society's Web site supplies information about obesity surgery, including the conditions that affect long-term success.

Institute of Medicine (IOM) of the National Academies
500 Fifth Street NW
Washington, DC 20001
Phone: 202-334-2352
Fax: 202-334-2158

Web site: http://iom.edu
E-mail: iomwww@nas.edu

The National Academy of Sciences (NAS), signed into being by President Abraham Lincoln in 1863, was mandated to "investigate, examine, experiment, and report upon any subject of science or art" (National Academies 2008) whenever called upon to do so by any department of the government. NAS eventually expanded to include the National Research Council (1916), National Academy of Engineering (1964), and Institute of Medicine (1970). Collectively, the organizations are known as the National Academies. IOM is a nonprofit organization whose present-day goal is to provide unbiased, science-based information concerning health policy to policy makers, professionals, and the public. It publishes reference values for nutrient intakes such as calories, carbohydrates, and fats, which are periodically updated.

The IOM, in conjunction with the Robert Wood Johnson Foundation, assessed the progress made in response to the 2005 IOM report *Preventing Childhood Obesity: Health in the Balance*. The report provided a guide with detailed actions for government, industry, media, communities, schools, and families for prevention and treatment of obesity in children and youth. The assessment report, *Progress in Preventing Childhood Obesity: How Do We Measure Up?* launched a call to action for key stakeholders to continue to monitor effectiveness of new policies and programs and to widely publicize the most promising practices. The IOM Web site includes published reports about obesity including such fact sheets as what the government, industry, and foundations can do to respond to childhood obesity. This page features links to current projects, many of which are devoted to the study of obesity in adults and children.

International Food Information Council (IFIC)
1100 Connecticut Avenue NW, Suite 432
Washington, DC 20036
Phone: 202-296-6540
Web site: http://ific.org
E-mail: foodinfo@ific.org

IFIC provides information on food safety, nutrition, and health to health professionals, educators, journalists, and government officials who are responsible for relaying this information to the public. They examine the latest research and break it down into understandable information for consumers. The IFIC media guide on food safety and nutrition lists experts and their contacts in a number of different specialties.

IFIC is supported by the food, beverage, and agricultural industries. It produces a bimonthly newsletter on current topics in food safety and nutrition. The IFIC Web site has resources that are understandable and useful for consumers and health professionals. It contains a glossary of food-related terms, brochures and fact sheets, videos on current health topics, and a newsroom filled with the latest health information. IFIC developed a partnership with America on the Move, the Food Marketing Institute, and the President's Council on Physical Fitness and Sports to create Kidnetic. This is a Web site program for kids and their parents to learn about nutrition and health in a fun and interactive way. It provides kid-friendly recipes, games, and physical activity ideas.

IFIC is based in Washington, DC, and focuses primarily on U.S. issues; however, it also contributes to an informal network of food information organizations in Europe, Asia, Australia, Canada, Japan, New Zealand, and South Africa.

National Association to Advance Fat Acceptance (NAAFA)
P.O. Box 22510
Oakland, CA 94609
Phone: 916-558-6880
Web site: www.naafa.org
e-mail: info@naafa.org

NAAFA works to eradicate stigma and discrimination based on body size. The tools used are public education, advocacy, and support for association members. It is a forum where issues affecting fat people can be discussed in an unbiased setting. NAAFA provides a legal aid program called FLARE (Fat Legal Advocacy, Rights, and Education) to help people facing size-related discrimination. NAAFA offers its members activities and opportunities to get more information and a chance to help the fight against size discrimination. The NAAFA newsletter has up-to-date listings of research, legal, and legislative issues and schedules for the Association's meetings and programs. The Fat Activist Task Force encourages letter-writing campaigns that protest or praise advertising and media targets that portray obese people. Local NAAFA chapters throughout the United States are led by volunteers and carry out NAAFA's mission at the local level. Most chapters hold local meetings and sponsor workshops and support groups. A wide range of special interest groups (SIGs) within NAAFA that provide programs for members sharing common concerns include Big Men's Forum, Couples SIG, Diabetic SIG, Military Issues SIG, and Weight Loss Surgery Survivors SIG. Each year NAAFA holds a national meeting that allows members from around the United States to network. These meetings present educational and social activities such as workshops, rallies, sightseeing trips, swim parties, and fashion shows.

Specific resources available on the NAAFA Web site include guidelines for health care providers, facts about hypertension, and myths about weight loss and fat people. Pamphlets are available for download on the following topics: "Airline Tips for Large Passengers," "Declaration of Health Rights for Fat People," and "Joining the Size Acceptance Revolution."

The Obesity Society (TOS)
8630 Fenton Street, Suite 814
Silver Spring, MD 20910
Phone: 301-563-6526
Web site: http://www.obesity.org/

Founded in 1982, TOS is the leading scientific society dedicated to the study of obesity. It supports obesity research, education, and advocacy. The organization publishes research on the causes and treatment of obesity, keeps the medical community and public informed of new advances, and aims to improve the lives of people with obesity. It publishes the journal*Obesity.*

In November 2004, TOS's Council developed a new strategic plan to expand and define the Society's focus. It is committed to advancing public policy changes that focuses on assessment, prevention, and treatment of obesity. TOS's advocacy program objectives include developing programs designed to prevent obesity, ensuring that all people have access to quality medical care for obesity treatment, and increasing funding for obesity research. In pursuing these objectives, he Obesity Society works with the U.S. Congress, the U.S. Surgeon General, and CDC. At the presidential nominating conventions in 2008, The Obesity

262 Directory of Agencies, Programs, and Organizations

Society presented a forum entitled "The Challenge of Obesity for Policy Makers: Recommendations for the Next Administration," which featured roundtable discussions with policy makers at both the national and local level, in addition to representatives of Barack Obama and John McCain, the Democratic and Republican Party nominees in the 2008 presidential election, respectively.

The Society has issued numerous position statements that represent the organization's official stance, such as "Guidance for Industry on Developing Products for Weight Management," "Position on Orlistat as an Over-the-Counter Drug," "National Coverage Determination for Bariatric Surgery," and "Comments on Medicare Policy." For consumers, the Web site offers fact sheets: "Obesity and Diabetes," "Obesity and Cancer," and "Childhood Overweight, Obesity, Bias, and Stigmatization" are some examples.

Robert Wood Johnson Foundation (RWJF)
Route One and College Road East
P.O. Box 2316
Princeton, NJ 08543-2319
Phone: 877-843-7953
Web site: http://www.rwjf.org
E-mail: http://www.rwjf.org/global/contactus.jsp

RWJF is a philanthropic organization devoted to improving health policies and practices. It works with individuals, universities, and organizations to address health problems at their roots. RWJF focuses on improving health care to help Americans lead healthier lives. The foundation acknowledged the obesity epidemic in the United States by declaring to help reverse it by 2015. Its strategies include investing in research to prevent obesity, action to bring about results, and advocacy to educate policy makers.

The RWJF childhood obesity prevention program offers funding for studies that test ways to improve childhood physical activity and nutrition. The Web site presents research results, such as one entitled "U.S. Secondary Schools Serving Up Unhealthy Foods." The study, published in the journal *Pediatrics*, showed that the foods and food policies in U.S. public schools become less healthy as students progress from elementary to high school. The Foundation developed the Sports4Kids program, which enables kids to become more physically active at school through organized recreational activities at recess and after school. RWJF is working on bringing affordable and nutritious foods to urban areas nationwide by collaborating with the Philadelphia Food Trust advocacy organization.

Rudd Center for Food Policy and Obesity
309 Edwards Street
Yale University
New Haven, CT 06520-8369
Phone: 203-432-6700
Web site: yaleruddcenter.org/
E-mail: rudd.center@yale.edu

Founded in 2005, the Yale University Rudd Center for Food Policy and Obesity is a nonprofit research and public policy organization. Its global goals are to prevent obesity, improve dietary choices, and transform the way in which overweight and obese persons are viewed by the public. To pursue universal health changes, the Rudd Center interacts with the media, industry and government, and grassroots activists. The Center depends upon experts from around the world who represent varied opinions about obesity-related issues in science, law, business, and bioethics. It describes its work as being at the intersection of science and public policy. The Rudd Center's current research studies are designed to increase understanding of the factors that affect how we eat, how we discriminate against overweight and obese people, and how we can change.

Through its Web site, details of these studies and information about obesity are available to the general public, health care professionals, policy makers, schools, and educators. Podcasts, handouts, faculty presentations, and a free monthly newsletter are also some of the resources.

Shape Up America!
6707 Democracy Boulevard, Suite 306
Bethesda, MD 20817
Phone: 301-493-5368
Web site: http://www.shapeup.org
E-mail: http://www.shapeup.org/contact/contact_std1.php

Shape Up America! is a national initiative founded in 1994 by former Surgeon General C. Everett Koop to promote awareness of obesity as a major public health priority and to provide responsible information on healthy weight management. Its mission is based on the scientific evidence that obesity is a serious health condition and not just an appearance problem. The organization aims to increase cooperation among national and community organizations to make healthy weight and increased physical activity a possibility for all Americans. It seeks to educate the public on how to achieve a healthful weight through increased physical activity and healthy eating. The Shape Up America! Web site is designed to give information to the public, health care professionals, educators, and the media. The professional center contains tools and reports on obesity assessment, treatment, and monitoring. For individuals, there are interactive assessment tools, meal planning guides, and recipes. The *Parents Guide for the Assessment and Treatment of the Overweight Child* provides helpful information for a parent or caregiver of an overweight child on how to increase the chances of successful weight management. A key message is that treatment of childhood obesity should improve the lifestyle of the entire family and not just focus on the child. Ideas and tips for achieving that goal are included in the *Guide*.

Shaping America's Youth (SAY)
120 NW 9th Avenue, Suite 216
Portland, OR 97209-3326
Phone: 800-SAY-9221 (800-729-9221)
Fax: 503-273-8778
Web site: www.shapingamericasyouth.com
E-mail: info@shapingamericasyouth.com

SAY, founded by Kate and David McCarron, is an innovative effort to prevent and reduce childhood obesity. It holds town hall meetings to talk with parents and children to find out what information they want and need to create a community-based action plan. SAY's goal is to provide the latest and most comprehensive information on community efforts that are directed at improving the health of American youth.

Its Web site has an online survey to collect demographic and funding information about programs throughout the United States that strive to improve childhood nutrition and physical activity. SAY is a national clearinghouse for this collected information. The site also offers childhood obesity funding opportunities, publications, schedules of SAY Town Meetings, and other resources related to childhood obesity.

Trust for America's Health (TFAH)
1730 M St. NW, Suite 900
Washington, DC 20036
Phone: 202-223-9870
Fax: 202-223-9871
Web site: http://healthyamericans.org
E-mail: info@tfah.org

TFAH is a nonprofit, nonpartisan organization that works to make disease prevention a national priority. TFAH supports a strong and responsive public health system that is vital for preventing disease. On the Web site, the yearly Public Policy Priorities are set forth. Each year, TFAH produces a report on the national status of obesity entitled "F as in Fat: How Obesity Policies are Failing in America," which includes a review of federal and state obesity policies and obesity facts for each state. The "How Healthy Is Your State" drop-down menu for individual states includes obesity rates in adults and children, hypertension rates, diabetes rates, and percentage of adults who are physically inactive as well as per capita medical costs of obesity.

Veterans Administration National Center for Health Promotion and Disease Prevention
3022 Croasdaile Drive, Suite 200
Durham, NC 27705
Phone: 919-383-7874
Web site: www.healthierusveterans.va.gov
Contact: HealthierUSVeterans@va.gov.

In February 2006, the Department of Veterans Affairs (VA) and HHS launched an initiative called HealthierUS Veterans. Based on the presidential initiative HealthierUS, this initiative seeks to improve the health of veterans and their families across the country. A particular focus is placed on obesity and diabetes, as they are major health concerns for veterans and the VA health care system. The HealthierUS Veterans Web site features the My HealtheVet link, which offers tools for tracking food intake and physical activity. The toolkit on the Web site provides a guide for local and state-based VA agencies to implement programs such as The MOVE! Weight Management Program, a patient-centered plan to help veterans lose weight and keep it off. Other features on the Web site are brochures such as "Eat Healthy, Be Active and "Get Fit for Life," a virtual grocery store tour, and public service announcement video segments. Obesity prevention interventions that are ongoing in local VA agencies are listed on the Web site. For example, veterans can participate in the "Step Up to Your Health: Stair Use" promotion or a "Learn Healthier Cooking Skills for a Healthier You" class.

William J. Clinton Foundation (WJCF)
55 West 125th Street
New York, NY 10027
Web site: http://www.healthiergeneration.org/contact.aspx
E-mail: Info@HealthierGeneration.org

WJCF, in partnership with the American Heart Association and along with coleader Governor Arnold Schwarzenegger of California, has created the Alliance for a Healthier Generation. Its mission is to eliminate childhood obesity in the United States and to encourage young people to develop lifelong, healthy habits. To foster these changes, which can make a difference to a child's health, the Alliance calls upon schools, industry, health care, the community, and children themselves to make strides against obesity in the following ways.

The school programs focus on creating real, practical solutions to childhood weight management through healthier food choices and opportunities for activity in schools. The Foundation created the Healthy Schools Program and Kids Movement to put healthy foods and beverages in vending machines and cafeterias, to increase opportunities for students to exercise and play at school, and to provide resources for teachers and staff to become healthy role models. Through the industry programs, WJCF works with the food industry to persuade food purveyors, restaurants, and fast-food outlets to produce healthier drinks, snacks, and meals that are available to children. It is also helping the health care industry to better understand, diagnose, and treat childhood obesity.

The idea behind the Kids Movement plan was to motivate children to take charge of their health and to lead their own Go

Healthy movement. Details about the Let's Just Play Go Healthy Challenge, is found at http://www.nick.com/shows/lets_just _play/index.jhtml/. Nickelodeon and the American Heart Association teamed up with the William J. Clinton Foundation.

References

American Medical Association (AMA). Roadmaps for Clinical Practice series: Assessment and Management of Adult Obesity. 2007. [Online information; retrieved 1/12/09.] http://www.ama-assn.org/ama/pub/category/10931.html.

National Academies. "About the NAS." 2008. [Online information; retrieved 1/12/09.] http://www.nasonline.org/site/PageServer?pagename=ABOUT_main_page.

8

Selected Print and Nonprint Resources

This chapter offers a collection of resources in a variety of formats to help you get more specific or individualized information on the subject of obesity. Examples are provided from government agencies, nonprofit organizations, scientific experts, magazines, popular authors, and movie producers. This list is not all-inclusive, but it provides an inventory of obesity-related references, scientific and popular books, paper- and Web-based reports and guidelines, and journals and magazines that provide in-depth information about such areas as weight loss plans and scientific research. Another section includes newsletters that are helpful for keeping up-to-date about obesity prevention and management. Web sites developed by experts provide accurate information, statistics, and science. Interactive Web sites have practical tools to assess food choices. Motivational sites encourage physical activity and healthful eating with games, quizzes, and other interactive features that are meant to appeal to adults as well as children and teens. A list of movies is included that present interviews from some of America's experts in obesity, a look at the consequences of fast-food meals, and obesity stereotyping. Databases provide a range of information from the general to the scientific that can be useful for a further exploration of obesity in adults and children throughout the world. Finally, a list of calculators and counters aid in food measurement and keeping track of calories, body mass index (BMI), or childhood growth.

Books

Reference Works

2008 Health & Nutrition Yearbook. Editors of *Tufts Health & Nutrition Letter,* 2008, 200 pp. Publisher: D. B. Lee, *Tufts Health & Nutrition Letter.* Web site: http://www.tuftshealth letter.com/

The *2008 Health & Nutrition Yearbook* is based on a full year's content of the *Tufts Health & Nutrition Letter.* It is organized and indexed for easy reference. The book covers health topics like weight control, vitamins, sugar substitutes, antioxidants, and arthritis. Also included is a section titled "Ask Tufts Experts."

Alternative Sweeteners, Third Edition, Revised and Expanded. L. O'Brien-Nabors and Robert C. Gelardi. Marcel Dekker, Inc.; New York, 1991, 553 pp. ISBN: 0-8247-0437-1

The number of alternative sweeteners is large enough for O'Brien-Nabors and Gelardi to write a 553-page book about them. Each review of a sweetener is extensive. For example, the chapter on sucralose is 22 pages long. This third edition includes numerous new types of sweeteners. These individual reviews include scientific information, technical applications, and regulatory ratings. Sweeteners are compared with sucrose (table sugar). Many of the sweeteners have fewer calories than sucrose. The authors work for the Calorie Control Council, a nonprofit organization funded by industry.

Handbook of Nutraceuticals and Functional Foods. Robert E. C. Wildman. CDC Press, Taylor & Francis Group, 2007, 541 pp. ISBN 0-8493-6409-4

This authoritative handbook has 28 review articles written by experts. The underlying premise is that people can make their diet more healthful by adding dietary supplements or foods that have been formulated or fortified to include health-promoting factors. Several chapters discuss obesity, including one that covers using protein as a functional food ingredient for weight loss.

Scientific Works

The China Study. Colin T. Campbell and Thomas M. Campbell II. Dallas: Benbella Books, Inc., 2006, 417 pp. ISBN: 1-932100-66-0

Collin T. Campbell, professor emeritus at Cornell University, and Thomas M. Campbell II are both graduates of Cornell. They wrote this book based on research they conducted in a 20-year project in partnership with Cornell, Oxford University, and the Chinese Academy of Preventive Medicine that examined the lifestyle factors and diseases of 65 rural parts of China and Taiwan. This study was termed "The China Study," and it reported more than 8,000 statistically significant associations between lifestyle, diet, and disease variables. This book examines the associations discovered through this study. Issues discussed include the diseases of affluence (obesity, heart disease, cancer, and diabetes), how to eat, and why this information has not yet been publicized.

Obesity. Elliott M. Blass. Sunderland, MA: Sinauer Associates, Inc., 2008. 457 pp. ISBN-13: 978-0-87893-209-2

Elliott M. Blass is an expert in the field of obesity. In this book he brought together experts from different areas of obesity such as epidemiology, gastrointestinal physiology, drug addiction, exercise science, and agricultural policy to write chapters that represent all fields related to obesity. Examples of chapters include "Environmental Food Messages and Childhood Obesity" and "Exercise for Obesity Treatment and Prevention: Current Perspectives and Controversies."

Progress in Obesity Research: 8. Bernard Guy-Grand and Gerard Ailhaud. London: John Libbey & Co, Ltd. 1999, 864 pp. ISBN: 0-86196-581-7

The International Congress on Obesity is sponsored by the International Association (IASO). Internationally known experts on obesity gather every four years to discuss recent advancements in the field. This book presents topics that formed the basis of presentations from the 1998 meeting in Paris. This meeting was the first international congress of the "leptin era" and the last congress of the millennium. In the foreword, the editors wrote, "Most importantly, we do hope that these Proceedings will represent a landmark in getting all policy makers to consider the obesity epidemic very seriously by taking into account the thorough work of the International Obesity Task Force publicized by the World Health Organization. In this respect, the food and agricultural industry should play an increasing role in preventing this epidemic in developed and developing countries." In the decade since the publication of this reference book, the global epidemic has gotten much worse.

Progress in Obesity Research: 9. G. Medeiros-Meto, A. Halpern, and Claude Bouchard. Montrouge John Libbey Eurotext Ltd., 2003, 1080 pp. ISBN: 2-7420-0406-2

This is another in the series of books based on the conferences of the International Association for the Study of Obesity. This meeting was held in 2002 in Sao Paulo, Brazil. The chapters range from basic information to applied research. Chapters cover the international perspective on obesity drug therapy, the roles of behavior modification in the management of obesity, and an evaluation of the costs of obesity.

Popular Books

These are examples of popular diet books. Listing a book does not mean that it is an approved diet. Some fad diets are included here to aid in identifying false claims. Check the Federal Trade Commission report listed in this chapter, entitled *Weight Loss Advertising*. It provides criteria for evaluation of diets and claims.

The Alternative Day Diet: Diet Only Half the Time. James B. Johnson. G. P. Putnam's Sons, 2008, 288 pp. ISBN-13: 978-0-399-15493-5

The diet approach described in *The Alternative Day Diet* is a modified fast. No foods are off limits. The "down days" are days on which dieters must limit themselves to 300 to 500 calories. For the down days in the first few weeks, dieters are advised to sip protein shakes throughout the day. This is a classic fad that overpromises weight loss. One claim is that this diet will turn on a "skinny gene" to help the user shed the pounds and live a longer life. The author is a plastic surgeon.

Don't Eat This Book: Fast Food and the Supersizing of America. **Morgan Spurlock. Berkeley, CA: Penguin, 2005, 320 pp. ISBN-10: 0399152601**

After filming his movie *Super Size Me*, Morgan Spurlock wrote this book to summarize the conclusions of his 30-day McDonald's fast-food diet. He discusses why he believes so many Americans are obese today. It includes details of interviews he held with law officials, marketing professionals, and obesity experts.

Eat, Drink, and Be Healthy: The Harvard Medical School Guide to Healthy Eating. **Walter C. Willett, MD, and Patrick J. Skerrett. New York: Free Press, 2001, 348 pp. ISBN-10: 0743266420**

Eat, Drink, and Be Healthy is codeveloped with the Harvard School of Public Health. This book sorts through diet myths and explains how weight control is one of the single most important health benefits. Chapters include "Carbohydrates for Better and Worse" and "Surprising News about Fat and Healthy Weight." Also included are menu plans and recipes to make choosing the right foods easy.

Ending the Food Fight: Guide Your Child to a Healthy Weight in a Fast Food/Fake Food World. **David Ludwig and Suzanne Rostler. New York: Houghton Mifflin, 2007, 352 pp. ISBN-10: 0547053681**

David Ludwig is a pediatrician and an endocrinologist at Children's Hospital in Boston and the director of the Optimal Weight for Life (OWL) program, which helps treat children who are overweight or obese. Suzanne Rostler is a dietitian at the OWL clinic. They collaborated on this book to give parents advice on how to help their children who have unhealthy weight. This book includes topics such as eating to feel full and getting physical. A nine-week program with 50 recipes and shopping lists is outlined.

Fast Food Nation. Eric Schlosser. New York: HarperCollins, 2001, 416 pp. ISBN-10: 0-06-083858-2

Journalist Schlosser, in *Fast Food Nation*, takes an inside look at the fast-food industry. He has been investigating the industry for years, and he discusses what he has found in great detail in this book, including how it has created the obesity epidemic, insight on how the food is prepared and produced, and how the industry targets our younger population through advertising. Some of the chapters are titled "Why the Fries Taste So Good," "On the Range, What's in the Meat," and "The American Way."

Fat Families, Thin Families: How to Save Your Family from the Obesity Trap. Amy Hendel, PA. Dallas: Benbella Books, Inc., 2008, 475 pp. ISBN-10: 9781933771496

Amy Hendel is a physician assistant, journalist, and health television correspondent. Her book is aimed at being a guide for families who want a healthier lifestyle. Topics include healthy rules for shopping, avoiding emotional eating, practical tips on how to make healthy choices, and recipes even for busy schedules.

Fat Land: How Americans Became the Fattest People in the World. Greg Critser. New York: Houghton Mifflin, 2002, 256 pp. ISBN-10: 0618164723

Greg Critser explains how the United States came to be overwhelmingly obese by using examples of the effects of class, politics, culture, and economics. As a past overweight American himself, he is able to provide an inside look at the challenges associated with being overweight. Chapters included are "Supersize Me," "What the Extra Calories Do To You," and "What Can Be Done."

Food Fight. Kelly D. Brownell, PhD, and Katherine B. Horgen, PhD. New York: McGraw-Hill, 2004, 356 pp. ISBN-13: 9780071438728

This book, written by Yale University's Brownell and Horgen, looks at how we live in a "toxic environment" when it comes to dietary health. It explores the factors that have created an increase in disease and an expanded waistline in the United States. *Food Fight* includes an explanation on how the unhealthful environment was created, what allows it to exist in our society, and what steps need to be taken to improve it.

Food Politics. **Marion Nestle, PhD, MPH. Berkeley, CA: University of California Press, 2002, 457 pp. ISBN-13: 9780520254039**

Food Politics, written by New York University Professor Marion Nestle, takes an inside look at how food companies' main goal of selling more product and getting consumers to eat more affects our health. Points covered include ways that food companies undermine dietary advice and how kids and schools are exploited.

Good Calories, Bad Calories: Challenging the Conventional Wisdom on Diet, Weight Control, and Disease. **Gary Taubes. New York: Alfred A. Knopf, 2007, 601 pp. ISBN-13: 9781400040780**

Gary Taubes is a science writer. This book explores how the types of foods we consume are the key link to health. Emphasis is focused on the roles of fat and cholesterol, the roles of carbohydrates, and how these nutrients affect obesity and weight regulation.

Mayo Clinic on Healthy Weight. **Donald D. Hensrud, MD, Editor-in-Chief. Rochester, MN: Mayo Clinic, 2000, 200 pp. ISBN-10: 1-893005-05-4**

This book does not lay out a weight-loss diet, but it does provide the information that the physicians and dietitians at the famous Mayo Clinic give patients about weight control. The nondiet approach provides realistic guides for getting motivated and meal planning. It is well organized with informative headings and illustrated with helpful charts.

Mindless Eating: Why We Eat More Than We Think. **Brian Wansink, PhD. New York: Bantam Dell, 2006, 276 pp. ISBN-13: 9780553384482. ISBN-13: 9780739340370 (compact disc)**

Brian Wansink is a professor at Cornell University who has spent time at the U.S. Department of Agriculture (USDA). *Mindless Eating* examines the variables that cause one to consume food. Topics include the marketing of foods, environmental cues that influence our eating behavior, experiments that look at dietary decisions, and how to "mindlessly eat better."

Tyler's Honest Herbal, 4th Edition. **Steven Foster and Varro E. Tyler. Haworth Press, 1999, 442 pp. ISBN-10: 0-7890-0705-3**

A number of dietary supplements for weight loss contain herbs or herbal extracts. *The Honest Herbal* was originally published in the late 1970s. It continues to be the most referenced, quoted, and controversial book on herbs. Varro Tyler is distinguished professor emeritus at Purdue University. The authors write that herbs can make a significant positive contribution to health but that scientific studies need to be done to show how, and if, the herbs can be effective for weight loss.

The Volumetrics Eating Plan: Techniques and Recipes for Feeling Full on Fewer Calories. **Barbara J. Rolls. New York: HarperCollins, 2005 (trade paper), 2007; 317 pp. ISBN-13: 978-0-06-073730-6**

The Volumetrics Eating Plan, by Pennsylvania State University professor and researcher Barbara J. Rolls is a companion to *Volumetrics: Feel Full on Fewer Calories.* It provides strategies and easy-to-prepare recipes designed to help people eat more slowly and feel full on fewer calories.

The Volumetrics Weight-Control Plan: Feel Full on Fewer Calories. **Barbara J. Rolls and Robert A. Barnett. New York: Harpertorch, 2003, 369 pp. ISBN-10: 0-380-82117-6**

Professor Rolls, a well-respected researcher on food intake and weight management, and Robert A. Barnett, a nationally known food writer, collaborated on this book, which shows how to eat enough food to be satisfied, meet nutritional needs, and still lose weight. The volumetrics plan is developed from studies about the science of satiety and what researchers have learned about the food choices that make people feel full. The authors teach how to eat low-calorie-dense, high-volume foods to feel full even while eating fewer calories. The emphasis is on developing lifelong healthy eating skills. Some of the foods featured are hot soups (they have to be eaten slowly) and large salads. Recipes and meal plans are included.

What to Eat: An Aisle-by-Aisle Guide to Savvy Food Choices and Good Eating. **Marion Nestle, PhD, MPH. New York: North Point Press, 2006, 611 pp. ISBN-13: 9780865477049**

This book is written by Professor Marion Nestle from New York University. With all the confusion about what to eat or how to shop for the most healthful foods, *What to Eat* provides a step-by-step guide on how to make the best of a supermarket visit. The book explores each section of a typical supermarket and explains in common language ways to avoid the label confusion associated with shopping.

Women Afraid to Eat: Breaking Free in Today's Weight-Obsessed World. **Frances M. Berg. Hettinger, ND: Healthy Weight Network, 2001, 380 pp. ISBN-10: 0-918532-62-0**

Women Afraid to Eat provides an overview of current social and medical pressures to be thin. True stories of women illustrate the consequences of weight loss and dieting and the effects of starvation. The observations are backed up with research and statistics. The author devotes the second half of her book to suggestions on how women can be healthy no matter what their weight. She calls for changes in our weight-obsessed society and in the way overweight women are treated and asks for acceptance of all sizes. The information in the book is useful for health professionals, parents, coaches, and anyone who is concerned about women's health.

Reports

CDC Growth Charts: United States. **National Center for Health Statistics. http://www.cdc.gov/growthcharts**

By plotting height and weight measurements on an appropriate age-and-gender-specific growth chart, health care providers can monitor growth and identify potential health- or nutrition-related problems in children. Most of the data used to construct these charts come from the National Health and Nutrition Examination Survey (NHANES), which has collected height and weight information on the American population since the early 1960s. In 2000 the CDC released new growth charts for children. The CDC charts replace the older versions of charts for children's height and weight based on data organized in 1977 since children are taller and heavier these days. By using these charts you can compare growth in infants from birth, children, and adolescents to age 20 with a nationally representative reference population based on young people of all ages and racial or ethnic groups.

Childhood Obesity: Harnessing the Power of Public and Private Partnerships. **S. Maelpati, H. Pirani, D. Surie, D. Dietz. J. Lee. National Institute for Health Care Management Foundation. 1225 19th St., NY Suite 710. Washington, DC 20036. Web site: http://www.NIHCM.org**

In this report the National Institute for Health Care Management Foundation (NIHCM) highlights some outstanding collaboration between state health agencies and private health plans to reduce overweight and obesity in children. The NIHCM Foundation mission is to encourage cooperation between the public and private sectors to find creative solutions to American health care system problems. The report profiles cases of partnerships in Massachusetts, Pennsylvania and Tennessee and North Carolina. The report identifies eight vital components that interact to form a coordinated school health approach. These include: 1. Health education. 2. Physical education. 3. Health services. 4. Nutrition services. 5. Counseling and psychological services. 6. Healthy school environment. 7. Health promotion for staff. 8. Family and community involvement.

Comprehensive Report on 2000 Growth Charts. **Series Report 11, Number 246. 2000. 201 pp. PHS 2001-1695. Web site: http://www.cdc.gov/growthcharts/**

This comprehensive report from the CDC contains the database used for the 2000 CDC pediatric growth charts for boys and girls. The methodologies used and detailed statistical presentations are included in this expanded report. Differences between the 1977 and the 2000 growth charts are illustrated, and users are shown how to make the transition to using the 2000 CDC Charts. These charts may be used by health care workers and researchers interested in surveillance, food assistance, and other activities that rely on following the growth of infants, children, and adolescents in the United States.

Dietary Reference Intakes: The Essential Guide to Nutrient Requirements. **J. M. McGinnis, Chair. Food and Nutrition Board of the Institute of Medicine and Health Canada. Washington, DC: National Academies Press, 2006, 560 pp. ISBN-10: 0-309-10091-7**

This report from the National Academies is a summary of eight volumes combined in one reference volume. It is organized by nutrient and reviews the function of each nutrient, its food sources, and recommendations for people for maintenance of health and reduction of risk of chronic diseases such as cardiovascular disease (CVD) and some cancers. It describes the estimated average requirements by gender and age. It also gives estimates as to tolerable upper levels to avoid toxicity of some nutrients.

F as in Fat: How Obesity Policies are Failing in America. **J. Levi, L. M. Segal, and E. Gadola. 1707 H Street NW, 7th Floor. Washington, DC: Trust for America's Health, 2008, 144 pp. Web site: http:// www.rwjf.org/files/research/fasinfat2007.pdf**

This is the fourth annual edition of *F as in Fat*. It is a report about the weaknesses of current policies and the need to develop "grand scale changes" to address the obesity crisis. Some of the federal and state policies examined include school nutrition and physical activity requirements, community approaches (e.g., snack taxes, smart growth community design initiatives), and other public health programs. Updates are provided on obesity-related state and federal legislation and initiatives. Results from an experts survey and a public opinion survey are presented. The recommendations are targeted at different stakeholders and consist of the following: (1) schools and school districts should take responsibility for feeding students well; (2) employers should have healthier work environments; (3) the food, beverage, and marketing industries should provide consistent nutrition labeling based on product size; and (4) the federal government should update agricultural policy to encourage healthy eating and revise the Food Pyramid so that it is less confusing.

Food Marketing to Children: Threat or Opportunity? J. M. McGinnis, J. A. Gootman, and V. I. Kraak, Editors. Washington, DC: National Academies Press, 2006, 536 pp. ISBN-10: 0-309-09713-4

This report is a comprehensive review of scientific publications in the area of the influence of marketing on nutritional beliefs, choices, practices, and outcomes for children and youth. Many of these advertised products are high in calories, fat, and sugar. Consumption of these foods is linked to childhood obesity.

Implementation of the WHO Global Strategy on Diet, Physical Activity and Health. WHO Consultation on Obesity. Geneva: World Health Organization, 1998, 276 pp. Web site: http://www.who.int/dietphysicalactivity/implementation/en/

Although this report was published in 1998, many of the concerns and challenges are current. It is a comprehensive report about the global public health problem of obesity. Data include global prevalence and trends, costs of overweight and obesity including health consequences, and health benefits and risks of weight loss. An interesting part of this report is the "What Has Been Done since 2004?" section, which shows what entire countries and concerned social and economic groups have done to implement this global strategy since its adoption by the WHO member states in May 2004.

Preventing Childhood Obesity: Health in the Balance. J. P. Koplan, C. T. Liverman, and V. A. Kraak, Editors. Washington, DC: National Academies Press, 2005, 436 pp. ISBN-10: 0-309-09196-9

This committee report from the National Academies examines the environmental, social, medical, and historical factors influencing childhood obesity. Because of the increase in childhood obesity throughout the United States, policy makers are encouraged to recognize it as one of the most critical public health threats today. The book offers a prevention-based action plan that identifies promising short-term and longer-term interventions. It also recommends roles that various sectors of society should play to find solutions to the growing problem.

Thought Leader Insight & Analysis: Obesity. **Dublin, Ireland: Research and Markets, 2008, 114 pp. Web site: http:// www.researchandmarkets.com/reports/604940/**

Thought Leader Insight & Analysis is based on interviews with seven anonymous, internationally recognized thought leaders. They determined that obesity is not treated like other chronic diseases such as diabetes and CVD. To quote the report, "The medical justification for treating obesity is not directly tied to hard outcomes and the pharmacoeconomics do not yet motivate 3rd-party payers to broadly reimburse for pharmacotherapies." The panel gave its perspectives on the "pipeline" of obesity drugs, efficacy, and side effects. The drugs evaluated included those that act in the brain as well as on the periphery and those that can promote food absorption. The online brochure is useful because it lists drugs and the manufacturers. The report is very expensive, at more than $6,000. It is not targeted to consumers.

Weight Loss Advertising. **R. L. Cleland, W. C. Gross, L. D. Koss, M. Daynard, and K. M. Muolo. Washington, DC: Federal Trade Commission, 2002, 40 pp + Appendix**

Weight Loss Advertising is a report by the Federal Trade Commission (FTC) with the Partnership for Healthy Weight Management, a coalition of representatives from science, academia, heath care professions, government, commercial enterprises, and organizations whose mission is to promote sound guidance on strategies for achieving and maintaining a healthy weight. The report concludes that false or misleading claims, such as exaggerated weight loss without diet or exercise, are widespread in advertisements for weight-loss products. The agency identified claims that should be rejected by responsible advertising outlets because, based on current scientific knowledge, they are impossible to accomplish. This report was the basis for an FTC education campaign that encourages the media to reject weight-loss product advertising on any product that contains any of the following seven false "red flag" claims:

Causes weight loss of 2 pounds or more a week for a month, or more without dieting or exercising

Causes substantial weight loss, no matter what or how much the consumer eats

Causes permanent weight loss even when the consumer stops using the product

Blocks the absorption of fat or calories to enable consumers to lose substantial weight

Safely enables consumers to lose more than 3 pounds per week for more than four weeks

Causes substantial weight loss for all users

Causes substantial weight loss by wearing it on the body or rubbing it into the skin

Guidelines

Clinical Guidelines on the Identification, Evaluation, and Treatment of Overweight and Obesity in Adults. **Bethesda, MD: National Heart, Lung and Blood Institute and National Institute of Diabetes and Digestive and Kidney Disease, 1998, 228 pp. Item No.: 98-4083. Web site: http://www.nhlbi.nih.gov/guidelines/obesity/ob_home.htm**

These are the first federal government guidelines to addresses obesity and overweight. The guidelines are evidence based using an extensive review of the scientific literature. They are written for health professionals who work with overweight and obese patients. The Preface (xvii) includes a table that displays the classifications for overweight and obesity by BMI; waist circumference; and associated disease risk for type 2 diabetes, hypertension, and CVD. For example, if one's BMI is between 30.0 and 34.9 (Class I Obesity) and waist circumference is ≤ 35 inches, disease risk is high. Females with a waist circumference of ≥ 35 inches and a BMI of 30.0–34.9 have a very high disease risk. Men with a waist circumference of ≤ 40 inches and ≥ 40 inches have a high and very high risk of disease, respectively. These parameters do not take into account physical activity.

Scientific evidence shows that one can have Class I Obesity and not be at high risk of other diseases, especially if physically fit.

Dietary Guidelines for Americans 2005. U.S. Department of Health and Human Services and U.S. Department of Agriculture. Alexandria, VA: USDA Center for Nutrition Policy and Promotion. Web site: htpp://www.health.gov /dietaryguidelines/dga2005/document/default.htm

The *Dietary Guidelines for Americans*, originally issued in 1980, is revised every five years. A committee is appointed by the secretaries of the U.S. Department of Health and Human Services (HHS) and USDA. The purpose of the guidelines is to provide science-based advice to promote health for Americans over two years of age. The 2005 guidelines placed stronger emphasis on reducing calorie consumption and increasing physical activity than did previous versions. The food and exercise plans for the *Dietary Guidelines* are graphically presented by the Food Guide Pyramid. The guidelines are intended for the public, policy makers, and nutrition educators. They can be downloaded from the Web site, along with the consumer brochure "Finding Your Way to a Healthier You."

Healthy People 2010 Initiative. Web site: www.healthy people.gov/

In January 2000, HHS launched Healthy People 2010, a comprehensive, nationwide health promotion and disease prevention agenda. It was designed to be a framework for improving the health of all people in the United States during the first decade of the 21st century. The promotion was built upon previous initiatives that had been proposed over the preceding two decades. The goals of increasing quality and years of healthy life and eliminating health disparities were broken down into objectives that would be used to measure progress. Each objective had a target to be achieved by the year 2010. Three targets directly related to obesity were to:

Increase the proportion of adults who are at a healthy weight to a target level of 60 percent of Americans

Reduce the proportion of adults who are obese to 15 percent

Reduce the proportion of children and adolescents who are
overweight or obese

Goals were set separately for each childhood age grouping,
with the overall reduction to be measured from a baseline of
11 percent to 5 percent of children and adolescents who are
overweight. By 2008, the United States had made little progress
toward those targets. In fact, the midcourse review indicated
that the obesity situation was getting worse. From this central
site, a number of other government Web sites can be accessed to
find information about obesity and weight control.

Journals and Magazines

Consumer Reports. **Consumers Union (CU). 1101 17th Street
NW Suite 500. Washington, DC 20036. Web site: http://
consumersunion.org**

Consumer Reports is published monthly by Consumers Union, a
nonprofit, independent testing and information organization. It
does not accept advertisements and thus is truly independent
and a reliable source of information. *Consumer Reports* has
reviewed weight-loss supplements and diets and diet programs. Searching its Web site by subject matter using the phrase
"weight loss diets" yields, for example, an article about banning
the sales of over-the-counter weight-loss products to people
under 18 in Florida. Also posted is a letter from CU editors that
calls for filing criminal charges against a company that uses
ephedra/ma huang in their products. Links are provided to
articles published in scientific journals.

International Journal of Obesity. **R. L. Atkinson and I.
Macdonald, Editors. Nature Publishing Group, London.
ISSN: 0307-0565; ESSN: 1476-5497. Web site: http://www
.nature.com/ijo. E-mail: c-zulkey@northwestern.edu**

The *International Journal of Obesity* is the official research journal
of the IASO, an organization that serves as an umbrella for 52
national obesity associations in 56 countries. The monthly
journal publishes research papers on basic, clinical, and applied
studies.

Journal of the American Dietetic Association. L. Van Horn, Editor. Elsevier Inc., Philadelphia, PA. ISSN 0002-8223. Web site: www.adajournal.org. E-mail: https://secure.nejm.org/ services/contactus/contact_home.aspx

The *Journal of the American Dietetic Association* is the official journal of the American Dietetic Association. It is a source for the practice and science of food, nutrition, and dietetics. It publishes original research articles, reviews, position papers, and abstracts of papers published in other journals. The journal publishes articles across a range of research and practice fields, such as medical nutrition therapy, public health nutrition, food science and biotechnology, food service systems, leadership and management, and dietetics education.

New England Journal of Medicine. J. M. Drazen, Editor. Massachusetts Medical Society. ISSN: 0028-4793. Web site: http://www.nejm.org

The *New England Journal of Medicine* is published weekly and is the official journal of the Massachusetts Medical Society. Articles are targeted to physicians and other health care professionals. It publishes primary research articles, review articles, and commentaries. It is an important source of medical news, including emerging information on obesity, and articles from new issues are often also reported in newspaper, radio, and television stories.

Nutrition Today. Johanna Dwyer, Editor-in-Chief. Lippincott Williams & Wilkins. ISSN: 0029-666X. Web site: http://www .nutritiontoday.com

Nutrition Today is published six times a year. It is primarily for nutritional professionals but is easy to read and valuable to consumers. It helps people clear a pathway through today's maze of fad diets and cure-all claims.

Obesity. R. N. Bergman, Editor-in-Chief. Nature Publishing Group, Cambridge, MA. ISSN: 1930-7381; EISSN: 1930-739X. Web site: http://www.obesity.org

Obesity (formerly known as *Obesity Research*) is the official research journal of The Obesity Society. It publishes research articles, review articles, commentaries, public health and medical developments, and abstracts from its annual meeting. It is published monthly.

Obesity Reviews. **A. Astrup, Editor. Blackwell Publishing. ISSN: 1467-7881. Web site: http://www.iaso.org**

Obesity Reviews, published bimonthly, is the official review journal of the IASO. Some reviews are available for free and can be downloaded. Examples of reviews include "Childhood Obesity: Are We Missing the Big Picture?" "International School-based Interventions for Preventing Obesity in Children," and "Fasting: The Ultimate Diet?"

Prevention. **Liz Vaccariello, Editor-in-Chief. Rodale, Inc. ISSN: 0032-8006. Web site: http://www.prevention.com**

Prevention magazine is published monthly. One focus of the publication is on maintaining good health. A number of articles, such as "Get a WOW BODY: Speed That Metabolism and Break That Plateau," are based on questionable notions. The articles are often written in a question-and-answer format. Its Web site offers several free *Prevention* newsletters, including "Eat Up, Slim Down" and "Walk Off Weight," as well as periodic news alerts. Many of its articles, while eye-catching, are not based on scientific evidence.

Newsletters

Berkeley Wellness Letter. **John Edward Swartzberg, Editorial Chair. University of California, Berkeley. ISSN (printed): 0748-9234**

The *Berkeley Wellness Letter* is a nutrition, fitness, and self-care newsletter published by the University of California, Berkeley. The newsletter has articles that support a positive, day-to-day approach to a healthful, active life. It includes both scientific and practical health guides from the latest research and conducts the most advanced tests to long-used home remedies and common sense. A goal for the newsletter's Web site is to develop a series of articles and fact sheets on the subjects of nutrition, longevity, and fitness, including "Guide to Dietary

Supplements," which will eventually be an online encyclopedia of wellness.

Consumers Magazines Digest. **Kristen McNutt, President of Consumer Choices Inc., Editor. Web site: http:// www.mcnuttwebsite.com**

This online newsletter is written by Kristen McNutt, president of Consumer Choices Inc. She is a professional nutrition communicator. The newsletter features stories about nutrition, food safety, functional foods, and health-related topics. The free newsletter is available electronically and is meant to be an education service for food and health professionals. The *Digest* reviews nutrition topics that appear in about 40 current U.S. and Canadian magazines. Some articles include "What Celebrity Success Stories Omit about Weight Loss Surgery" (*Glamour*), "People Underestimate the Calories in 'Junk'" (*Men's Health*), "Move It to Lose It" (*Good Housekeeping*), "Sleep Off the Pounds" (*Health*), Every Bit Helps" (*O Magazine*), "Scary Fair Food" (*Parents*), and "Weight Discrimination" (*Health*).

Nutrition Action Health Letter. **Center for Science in the Public Interest. 1875 Connecticut Ave. NW, Suite 300. Washington, DC 20009. Phone: 202-332-9110. Web site: http:// www.cspinet.org**

Nutrition Action Health Letter is published monthly by the Center for Science in the Public Interest, an advocacy organization for nutrition and health, food safety, alcohol policy, and sound science. This newsletter has about 900,000 subscribers in the United States and Canada. It periodically reviews fad diets and is usually a good source of information. The newsletter reports the results of studies it has conducted such as the calories and nutritional quality of restaurant meals and calorie labeling on menu boards of fast-food restaurant chains.

Nutrition Perspectives. **S. Zidenberg-Cherr, Editor. Department of Nutrition. University of California, Davis, CA 95616. Office: 530-752-3387. E-mail: szsidenbergcherr@ucdavis.edu**

Nutrition Perspectives is published bimonthly by the Department of Nutrition of the University of California, Davis. This newsletter summarizes the latest nutrition research and food-related programs (e.g., "Can Tomatoes Carry the Cure for Alzheimer's?"). Obesity research and programs are reviewed.

Shape Up America! Newsletter. **Barbara J. Moore, PhD, Editor-in-Chief. E-mail: newsletter@shapeup.org**

This newsletter is for consumers interested in learning more about obesity prevention and treatment. It features stories about people's weight-loss experiences. For example, the "My Story" section published an article about a man named Dennis who lost 85 pounds over five months. Following publication, a reader wrote to comment that she was disappointed to see an article about what she thought was unhealthy because so much weight was lost without medical supervision. The editor, Dr. Moore, replied that when very obese people (Dennis weighed 290 pounds) start a diet, the decrease in calories is significant. A large part of early weight loss is water weight and some protein and fat. Dennis had also stopped drinking alcohol, which contributed to the decrease in his caloric intake. Moore added that after the initial weight-loss period, weekly weight loss should be closer to 2 pounds. In addition to personal stories, some articles relate experiences in communities. For example, acknowledging the observation that almost one-half of people age 12–21 years do not participate in vigorous physical activity on a regular basis, the newsletter published a report about how to get kids to increase their physical activity via intramural sports programs and other after-school activities.

Tufts Health & Nutrition Letter. **D. B. Lee, Publisher. Web site: http://www.tuftshealthletter.com**

The *Tufts Health & Nutrition Letter* was started in 1983 by then Tufts University President Jean Mayer as an outreach program of Tufts University and the Friedman School of Nutrition Science & Policy. By calling upon experts from the areas of clinical nutrition, social and public policy, and biomedicine, *Tufts Health & Nutrition Letter*'s aim is to provide the trustworthy and scientifically authoritative health and nutrition advice that can directly improve consumers' health. The newsletter has covered weight control in articles including "What Does the Latest Research on Weight Mean to You?"

"Diet or Exercise, It's Calories That Count," and "Gut-Check Time: Why Belly Fat Poses Extra Risks". Articles appear about vitamins, sugar substitutes, antioxidants, and arthritis, and the newsletter features a section called "Ask Tufts Experts."

Web Sites

General Web Sites

Baylor College of Medicine. Web site: http://www.bcm.edu /cnrc/resources/hottopics.html#obesity

Baylor College of Medicine maintains a Web site containing information about childhood obesity. It lists reports such as, "Healthy Weight Initiative" (American Dietetic Association), "Is Dieting OK for Kids?" (Nemours Foundation), "Keeping Kids Healthy: Obesity, Nutrition & Physical Activity" (Center for Health and Health Care in Schools), and "Soft Drinks in Schools" (American Academy of Pediatrics).

Diabetes in Control. Dave Joffe, Editor-in-Chief. Steve Freed, Publisher. Web site: http://www.diabetesincontrol.com/ index.php. E-mail: diabetes@topica.email-publisher.com

This online newsletter for health care professionals contains current news on diabetes that can be helpful to consumers. A number of the articles are about obesity. Newsletters include summaries of research articles such as "Gastric Bypass Surgery Reverses Metabolic Syndrome and "Studies Question Health Benefit of Post-Exercise Meals." Live Webcasts can also be accessed at the Web site.

Healthy Living. Brooke Claxton Building. Ottawa, Ontario K1A 0K9. Web site: http://www.hc-sc.gc.ca/hl-vs/index-eng. php. E-mail: Info@hc-sc.gc.ca

Healthy Living is a Web site of Health Canada where articles such as "Obesity (It's Your Health)," "Risk Factors for Heart Disease," and Canada's Food Guide to Healthy Eating" may be accessed. The primary focus is promoting healthy eating and healthy weights. Also provided are links to other Canadian government sites that provide additional information about obesity.

International Food Information Council (IFIC). Web site: http://www.ific.org/nutrition/obesity/index.cfm

The International Food Information Council's Web site provides information on food safety and nutrition to health professionals, educators, journalists, and government officials who are responsible for relaying this information to the public. It includes a section titled "Overweight, Obesity & Weight Management," which examines the latest research and breaks it down into understandable information for the general public. Its Web site has resources such as a glossary of food related terms, brochures and fact sheets, videos on current health topics, and a newsroom filled with the latest health information. IFIC partners with America on the Move, Food Marketing Institute, and the Presidents Council on Physical Fitness and Sports to create a Web site, called Kidnetic, for kids and their parents to learn about nutrition and health in a fun and interactive way (http:/kidnetic.com). It provides recipes, games, and exciting ways to obtain physical fitness. IFIC is supported by the food, beverage, and agricultural industries.

MedlinePlus®. U.S. National Library of Medicine and National Institutes of Health. Web site: www.nlm.nih.gov/ medlineplus

This Web site has information for both health professionals and consumers. It contains extensive information from NIH and other trusted sources on more than 600 diseases and conditions. Available on the Web site are a medical encyclopedia and a medical dictionary, health information in Spanish, information on prescription and nonprescription drugs, health information from the media, and links to thousands of clinical trials.

Rudd Center for Food Policy and Obesity. Yale University. New Haven, CT. Web site: http://www.yaleruddcenter.org/

The Yale Rudd Center aims to draw attention to weight bias and prejudice. Its goal is to develop strategies to address the issue with young people, families, teachers, employers, and health care professionals. The Web site provides comprehensive lists of research articles, research tools, and PowerPoint presentations for educators, students, and researchers who are interested in studying weight bias. All the materials on this site may be downloaded for free.

Weight-control Information Network (WIN). National Institute of Diabetes and Digestive and Kidney Disease (NIDDK). 1 WIN Way. Bethesda, MD 20892-3665. Web site: http://win .niddk.nih.gov/publications/better_health.htm

WIN is an information service of NIDDK. Its focus is on providing information about body weight to the public and media. The coverage of WIN reports and articles ranges from underweight to normal weight to obesity. WIN provides information about risks associated with overweight and obesity with special emphasis on diabetes. *WIN Notes* is a quarterly newsletter for consumers and health professionals. Also available is a series of booklets in English and Spanish that cover topics such as what is a healthy weight, getting active and healthy eating, and physical activity across the life span. Some of these booklets can be downloaded from the Web site.

Interactive for General Population

MyPyramid Tracker. Web site: http://www.mypyramidtracker .gov/

MyPyramid Tracker allows the user to assess his or her diet and physical activity. This tool can automatically calculate energy intake by subtracting one's physical activity from the energy intake (food calories). This site translates the principles of the USDA and HHS *Dietary Guidelines for Americans* for the consumer. Other sites related to MyPyramid include MyPyramid for Preschoolers and MyPyramid Menu Planner.

Rethink Your Drink. Web site: http://www.cdc.gov/nccdphp/ dnpa/healthyweight/healthy_eating/drinks.htm

This Web site lists the calorie content in various beverages and suggests substitutions that will help to decrease calories. For example, a 20-ounce bottle of nondiet cola has 227 calories. The suggested replacement is a beverage with zero calories such as diet soda or water. Another recommendation is to substitute a 12-ounce medium café latte with whole milk, containing 265 calories, with the same drink using fat-free milk, with just 125 calories. Another section of the Web site covers portion sizes and calories, including learning how to read nutrition fact labels carefully.

Shape Up America! Cyberkitchen. Web site: http://www .shapeup.org/atmstd/kitchen/page0.php

Shape Up America! founded in 1994, is a national initiative to promote awareness of obesity as a major public health priority and to provide responsible information on healthy weight management. The organization's Cyberkitchen is an interactive guide to healthy eating and weight management and teaches the user how to balance the food eaten with physical activity. Clicking on "I'm new here; show me what to do" leads to a tailored approach based on one's nutrition needs and eating style. Based on age, height, weight, gender, and physical activity, an estimated calorie goal is provided that can be adjusted if the user wants to lose or gain weight. The site also allows monitoring of daily dietary fat using the fat grams calculator. Suggestions are made as to how to burn extra calories or add extra calories. Recipes and a shopping list based on meal choices can be generated. The site is easy to use and helps people plan in advance what to eat.

Treatment Guidelines Implementation Tool for Palm OS and PocketPC2003 Devices. Web site: http://hp2010.nhlbihin.net/ bmi_palm.htm

This tool is based on the NIH *Clinical Guidelines for Overweight and Obesity* and it is part of the Obesity Education Initiative at National Heart, Lung and Blood Institute. It is intended for health care professionals to use in patient care. Included is an automatic BMI calculator that can be downloaded to any handheld device that uses a Palm operating system.

Interactive for Children and Adolescents

BAM! Body and Mind Food & Nutrition. Web site: http:// www.bam.gov/sub_foodnutrition/index.html

BAM! Body and Mind is a resource developed for students by the Centers for Disease Control and Prevention that offers interactive content on health, safety, and science topics. Lessons are taught using games, challenges, and age-appropriate language. There is a section on energy, which reviews components of the kids' "energy equation": food + sleep + physical activity = energy. Users are prompted to think about the barriers to and benefits of acting on each component of the equation and develop a plan to put health knowledge into practice. The page entitled "Power Packing" describes how to pack tasty power lunches; "Fuel Up for Fun" has snack ideas to produce energy for physical activity; "Dining Decisions" is a game based on healthful food choices; and "Cool Treats" are recipes for quick and healthy snacks. The site also features success stories and an online calendar for tracking physical activity.

Eat Smart. Play Hard. Web site: http://www.fns.usda.gov/ eatsmartplayhardkids/

The Eat Smart. Play Hard. campaign was launched by the USDA's Food and Nutrition Service in 2000. This Web site encourages children and adults to eat healthful food and be physically active every day with kid-friendly, entertaining techniques. They can follow Power Panther, the campaign spokescharacter, and his nephew Slurp in exploring the Power Tunes Store, Theater, Fitness Center, Eat Smart Grill, Fun Times Arcade, and Travel Center. Behind each door in this virtual community is a location where everyone can learn healthy lifestyle skills through geography, music, reading, and science activities. All the resources on the site, including games and activities for children, brochures for parents, and educational tools for health professionals and educators, are consistent with messages from the *Dietary Guidelines for Americans* and the MyPyramid Food Guidance System.

Go With the Whole Grain for Kids Web site: http://www .bellinstitute.com/bihn/index.aspx?cat_1=83

This site provides worksheets, fact sheets, and a slide program. Grain Boy and Grain Girl, the energetic Whole Grain Heroes, explain what whole grains are, the benefits of eating whole grains, how to identify whole-grain foods, and how many servings of whole grains are recommended each day.

Kidnetic. International Food Information Council (IFIC). Web site: http://www.kidnetic.com/

Kidnetic is a Web site for kids and their parents to learn about the body, nutrition, and health in a fun and interactive way. It provides kid-friendly recipes, games, and exciting ways to obtain physical fitness. The International Food Information Council, an organization supported by food, beverage, and agricultural industries, has partnered with America on the Move, Food Marketing Institute, and the Presidents Council on Physical Fitness and Sports to create this Web site.

Media-Smart Youth: Eat, Think, and Be Active. Web site: http://www.nichd.nih.gov/msy/

Created by the Eunice Kennedy Shriver National Institute of Child Health and Human Development, the Media-Smart Youth program is an after-school program designed to help children learn about how to make smart food choices. It educates children on how the media can lead to poor health choices in their lives. Educating children about the media is important because many children spend hours watching television, playing video games, or surfing the web. All of these activities take time away from physical activity. They can lead to poor health choices based on the messages they display. This program is available to after-school providers or activity leaders for children to incorporate activities into their daily routines.

MyPyramid for Kids. Web site: http://mypyramid.gov/KIDS/

This Web site is designed for children 6 to 11 years old. It is the application of the *Dietary Guidelines for Americans* using MyPyramid. The site includes games, posters, worksheets to help kids track how their food choices match up to the recommendations of MyPyramid, tips for families, and classroom materials. One game, called "Blast Off," provides a "mission briefing" once the child enters his or her first name, age, and gender, which serves to "fuel up MyPyramid rocket ship with smart food choices and 60 minutes of physical activity to fly to Planet Power!" The target is 1,800 calories for the day. If, for example the child chooses a banana and yogurt for breakfast, that adds 270 food calories of fuel. The game is fun even if the user is older than 11 years old.

Nutrition Explorations. Web site: http://www.nutrition explorations.org

The National Dairy Council, a nonprofit organization, is supported by dairy producers. Its interactive Web site is for educators, parents, and kids. The kids' area of the Web site contains interactive games and activities, including "Fueled for Fun," "Monster Nutrition," and the Nutrition Tracker to record meals and check serving sizes. "Food Riddles" poses food-related jokes in form of riddles, such as the following:

Q: How do you make a strawberry shake?

A: You take it to a scary movie!

Q: What grain-group food do ghosts like for breakfast?

A: Scream of Wheat!

For educators, free school nutrition kits, nutrition expedition programs, and nutrition lessons are available. Parents may take advantage of back-to-school nutrition tips such as, "Jump start the day with breakfast." The "Ask the Expert" section allows people to ask questions.

Spot the Block: Get Your Food Facts First. Web site: http:// www.SpotTheBlock.com

To reach "tweens" (youth ages 9 to 13) in an effective and engaging way, the U.S. Food and Drug Administration is partnered with Time Warner's Cartoon Network to promote Spot the Block to tween audiences. Spot the Block is an educational campaign that encourages viewers to look for (spot) and use the nutrition facts (the block) before making food choices. The Cartoon Network features animated on-air spots, popular animated characters, and a Web site featuring the animated spots along with interactive nutrition messages and a nutrition label game. The two organizations are working together to prevent overweight and obesity in the early years, which can ultimately help young people stay healthy and prevent health problems in adulthood.

We Can! Ways to Enhance Children's Activity & Nutrition. Web site: http://www.nhlbi.nih.gov/health/public/heart/ obesity/wecan/

We Can! stands for Ways to Enhance Children's Activity & Nutrition. We Can! is a national education program of the National Heart, Lung and Blood Institute designed for parents and caregivers to help children 8–13 years old stay at a healthy weight. We Can! was launched in June 2005, and since that time schools, hospitals, parks and recreation departments, universities, private companies, and many other organizations have joined the movement. The goal of the We Can! partnerships is to build collaborations, preventive strategies, outreach efforts, and improved communication channels to circulate We Can! messages and materials to parents, caregivers, and youth ages 8–13 across the United States. Three behaviors are emphasized: improved food choices, increased physical activity and reduced screen time. We Can! is summarized by three phrases: learn it; live it, get involved. Links to individual sections are provided. Each section has background information and an action plan.

Movies

Fast Food Nation. **Date: 2006. Length: 106 min. Source: directed by Richard Linklater; executive producer Eric Schlosser Web site: http://www.fastfoodnationdvd.com**

Based on the book of the same title by Eric Schlosser, this film depicts the process of how the food served at fast-food restaurant chains reaches our plate. Processing, marketing, and the lives of those involved in the fast-food business are displayed in this film.

Killer at Large. **Date: 2008. Length: 106 min. Source: Shinebox Media Productions; produced by Bryan Young; directed by Neil LaBute. Web site: http://www.killeratlarge.com (content not yet available)**

This documentary film explores a variety of topics concerning the obesity epidemic in the United States. It provides interviews from some of America's experts and policy makers in obesity, including Richard L. Atkinson, Kelly Brownell, Dick Cheney, Bill Clinton, Michael Pollan, and former Surgeon General Richard Carmona. The film looks at school lunch and physical activity programs, media influences, lack of government programs, and what is being done to decrease the occurrence of obesity. It also examines specific examples of community initiatives, such as incorporating gardens in schools to teach children about food and nutrition. This movie explains causes, regulations, and possible solutions to the obesity epidemic in the United States.

The Nutty Professor. Date: 1996. Length: 96 min. Source: directed by Tom Shadyac; produced by Brian Grazer and Russell Simmons. Web site: http://www.nuttyprofessor.com

The Nutty Professor is a comedy film about a 400-pound professor of genetics, played by Eddie Murphy. The professor discovers a concoction that instantly sheds pounds. This movie provides an insight into the harsh stereotypes that go hand in hand with being overweight.

Super Size Me. Date: 2004. Length: 100 min. Source: Kathbur Pictures, Inc.; produced and directed by Morgan Spurlock. Web site: not available

Morgan Spurlock takes on the fast-food world by restricting his meals to only those foods available from McDonald's restaurants for 30 days in a row. His aim was to see if any health implications are associated with eating only fast food. As Spurlock embarks on this journey, he interviews obesity experts throughout the country to provide insight on the impact of the fast-food industry on the obesity epidemic in the United States.

Databases

CDC National Center for Chronic Disease Prevention and Health Promotion, Division of Nutrition and Physical Activity. Web site: http://www.cdc.gov/NCCDPHP/DNPA/

This Internet-based, searchable directory presents information on physical activity programs involving state departments of health. It is searchable by state and other key categories and includes brief program descriptions with information about partner organizations, status, scope, target population, setting, purpose, program components, evaluation, and products.

Contact information for programs within each state is also provided.

Combined Health Information Database (CHID). National Institutes of Health, Centers for Disease Control and Prevention. Web site: http://www.cehn.org/cehn/resourceguide/chid.html

CHID is a bibliographic database that displays titles, abstracts, books, fact sheets, and health information and health education resources. CHID provides a lists of a wealth of health promotion, education, and audiovisual materials as well as program descriptions that are not indexed elsewhere.

Economic Research Service (ERS). 1800 M Street NW. Washington, DC 20036-5831. Web site: http://www.ers .usda.gov/

ERS is part of the U.S. Department of Agriculture. Its mission is to be the primary source of economic information and research in the United States. With respect to obesity, data are gathered to study obesity, including the food supply and eating patterns.

International Bariatric Surgery Registry (IBSR). University of Iowa. Web site: http://www.healthcare.uiowa.edu/surgery/ibsr/

The purpose of IBSR is to promote the best care for patients who are having surgical treatment for severe obesity. IBSR is a centralized database of clinical research information for physicians with an interest in patient outcomes and assessment of medical treatment effectiveness. Results are used to study patient selection, practice variation, and surgical techniques in the treatment of obesity.

MedlinePlus®. Web site: http://medlineplus.gov/. U.S. National Library of Medicine and National Institutes of Health

This Web site directs both professionals and consumers to up-to-date, authoritative information about health questions. It contains details drawn from the world's largest medical library, the National Library of Medicine, on more than 600 diseases and conditions. It also has links to a medical encyclopedia, a medical dictionary, a drug/herbal index, and extensive information on prescription and nonprescription drugs. A news service for medical news reports is updated daily, and links to thousands of clinical trials are provided. Many of the links give health information in Spanish.

National Center for Health Statistics (NCHS). 3311 Toledo Road. Hyattsville, MD 20782. Web site: http://www.cdc.gov/nchs

NCHS, the United States' health statistics agency, compiles statistical information to guide actions and policies to improve the health of Americans as well as to serve as a public statistics resource on health topics including overweight prevalence, exercise and physical activity, nutrition, and diet. NCHS uses a number of different sources (e.g., birth and death records, medical records, interview surveys, direct physical exams, laboratory testing) to gather information about health issues. Results are presented in various simple and complex formats. For example, Data Briefs take a complex data subject and summarizes it into text and graphics that are easy to comprehend. Health Data Interactive presents tables with more complex national health statistics that can be customized by age, gender, race/ethnicity, and geographic location to explore different trends and patterns.

National Weight Control Registry (NWCR). Phone: 800-606-NWCR (6927). Web site: http://www.nwcr.ws

The NWCR was developed by Rena R. Wing and James O. Hill. Their research study has developed this database of people who have been successful at long-term maintenance of substantial weight loss. The registry includes people who are 18 years or older who have lost at least 30 pounds and have maintained a weight loss of at least 30 pounds or more. Enrollees are periodically asked to complete questionnaires about their success at losing weight, current weight maintenance strategies, and other health-related behaviors. NWCR members have lost an average of 66 pounds and kept it off for 5.5 years. Weight losses range from 30 to 300 pounds, and the duration of successful weight loss ranges from 1 to 66 years. Common strategies include the following: (1) 78 percent eat breakfast every day; (2) 75 percent weigh themselves at least once a week; (3) 62 percent watch less than 10 hours of TV per week; and (4) 90 percent exercise, on average, about one hour per day. The registry provides links to published scientific journal articles describing the eating and exercise habits of NWCR participants who have successfully lost weight, the behavioral strategies they use to maintain their weight, and the effect of successful weight-loss maintenance on other areas of their lives.

Nutrition.gov. Web site: http://www.nutrition.gov

The nutrition.gov Web site is managed by the staff at the Food and Nutrition Information Center (FNIC). FNIC has a staff of trained nutrition professionals, most of whom are registered dietitians, who provide science-based guidance on food and nutrition and are available to answer food and nutrition questions online. Specialized nutrition information is provided about infants, children, teens, adult women and men, and seniors.

Some of the topics include practical information on dietary supplements, fitness, and how to keep food safe. The site has the latest nutrition news and features links to interesting sites. The Web site also has links to all online federal government information about nutrition, healthy eating, physical activity, and food safety. Many of these resources are in Spanish.

**U.S. Physical Activity Statistics. Web site: http://apps.nccd
.cdc.gov/PASurveillance/StateSumV.asp**

This site provides information about prevalence of people in each state meeting physical activity recommendations. In 2007, less than 40 percent of the population of two states, Louisiana and Mississippi, met the requirements, and more than 50 percent of the population of nine states met the requirements (Alaska, Idaho, Maine, Montana, Oregon, Utah, Vermont, Wisconsin, and Wyoming). In 2001, more than 50 percent of people in 16 states met the requirements (Alaska, Arizona, Colorado, Hawaii, Idaho, Massachusetts, Maine, Montana, New Hampshire, New Mexico, Oregon, Utah, Vermont, Washington, Wisconsin, and Wyoming). Data may be retrieved for an individual state broken down by age groups from 18 to 65+.

WHO Global InfoBase. Web site: http://www.who.int/bmi/ index.jsp

The Global Database on Body Mass Index is an interactive surveillance tool for monitoring BMI around the world. The database displays adult underweight, overweight, and obesity prevalence rates by country, year of survey, and gender. The database is updated daily and has a search function that allows users to customize a data search that provides maps, tables, graphs, and downloadable documents. Obesity rates can be compared between chosen countries to highlight the scale of this global epidemic.

In June 2007, the World Health Organization launched a remodeled version of the Global InfoBase that is viewer friendly, is easy to navigate, and makes country data easily accessible. The WHO Global InfoBase contains reports on 180 out of 192 WHO member states, contains more than 130,000 data points from more than 2,800 sources, and allows each record to be linked back to all its survey information, including the primary source.

Food and Nutrition Experts

Calculators and Counters

Adult Energy Needs and BMI Calculator. Agricultural Research Service, USDA/ARS Children's Nutrition Research Center. Web site: http://www.bcm.edu/cnrc/caloriesneed.htm

To use this online calculator, enter the sex, height, weight, age, and activity level (about 20 to 50 percent of your calorie needs are determined by physical activity) to get one's BMI and calories needs per day to maintain current weight.

Body Fat Lab, Shape Up America! Web site: http://www .shapeup.org/bodylab/frmst.html

The Body Fat Lab provides a tool to determine percentage of body fat and its role in overall health. BMI can be calculated at this interactive Web site.

"Body Mass Index Table." National Heart, Lung and Blood Institute. Web site: http://www.nhlbi.nih.gov/guidelines/obesity/bmi_tbl.htm

This table shows BMI by seeing where one's height and body weight intersect on the chart. A version is also available to download and print.

The Calorie Counter, 4th Edition. Annette B. Natow, Ph.D., and Jo-Ann Heslin, M.A., R.D. New York: Pocket Books, 2007, 688 pp ISBN-10: 1-4165-0982-8

The Calorie Counter provides nutrition information such as calories, fat, protein, carbohydrates, and other nutrients for items at chain restaurants and for take-out foods. It also lists brand name foods found in grocery stores, energy bars and drinks, and ethnic foods. This book is small and easy to carry while shopping or dining out, and it contains more than 20,000 listings.

USDA National Nutrient Data Laboratory. Web site: http://www.ars.usda.gov/ba/bhnrc/ndl

The USDA National Nutrient Data Laboratory is a comprehensive tool for evaluating the nutritional value of 7,519 foods. These USDA databases are the foundation of most public and commercial nutrient databases used in the United States and a number of foreign countries. In addition, these data are used by food companies, trade associations, and research institutions.

Glossary

adipocytes   Fat cells.

adipose tissue   Fat tissue in the body.

anorexiant   A drug, a process, or an event that leads to anorexia, or lack of appetite.

appetite   Feelings of hunger and desire to eat.

bariatric   Pertaining to bariatrics, the field of medicine concerned with obesity and weight loss.

bariatric surgery   Also known as gastrointestinal surgery; surgery on the stomach and/or intestines to help patients with extreme obesity to lose weight.

BIA   Bioelectrical impedance analysis; a way to estimate the amount of body weight that is fat and nonfat by measuring the speed of a low-level electrical current as it moves through the body.

blood glucose   Glucose in the blood stream; blood sugar.

BMI   Body mass index; relates an individual's weight relative to his or her height. BMI is a person's weight in kilograms (kg) divided by his or her height in meters (m) squared. It also can be calculated by multiplying weight in pounds by 703 and then dividing that number by the individual's height in inches squared. The easiest way to figure BMI is to look it up in a table.

calipers   A metal or plastic tool similar to a compass used to measure the diameter of an object. The skinfold thickness in several parts of the body can be measured with skin calipers to determine the lean body mass.

calorie A unit of energy in food. Calories in foods may come from carbohydrates, proteins, fats, and alcohol. Carbohydrates and proteins have 4 calories per gram. Fat has 9 calories per gram. Alcohol has 7 calories per gram.

carbohydrate Carbohydrates have 4 calories per gram. Simple carbohydrates are sugars. Complex carbohydrates include both starches and fiber. Carbohydrates are found naturally in foods such as breads, pasta, cereals, fruits, vegetables, and milk and dairy products.

central fat distribution or abdominal fat Waist circumference is an index of body fat distribution. In android type (apple shaped) patterns, fat is deposited around the waist and upper abdominal area and appears most often in men. The gynoid type (pear shaped) distribution of body fat is usually seen in women. The fat is deposited around the hips, thighs, and buttocks.

childhood (pediatric) obesity See childhood overweight. (Though the term "childhood obesity" is commonly used, most health care providers refrain from using the term "obesity" in relation to children and adolescents. Instead, the condition is referred to as "overweight.")

childhood overweight The condition of children whose weight ranks above the 95th percentile of body mass index for age.

comorbidities Two or more diseases or conditions existing together in an individual.

CVD Cardiovascular disease; a disease of the heart or blood vessels; any abnormal condition characterized by dysfunction of the heart or blood vessels.

DEXA Dual energy X-ray absortiometry; a method used to estimate total body fat and percentage of body fat.

dexfenfluramine A weight-loss drug in a class of drugs called anorectics that decreases appetite. This drug, sold in the United States under the brand name Redux, was withdrawn from the U.S. market in 1997 because of its association with heart valve dysfunction.

diabetes Any of several metabolic disorders marked by increased blood glucose, excessive discharge of urine, and persistent thirst.

diastolic blood pressure   The minimum pressure that remains within the artery when the heart is at rest.

diet   What a person eats and drinks, or any type of eating plan.

energy balance   The state in which the total energy intake equals total energy needs.

energy deficit   The state in which total energy intake is less than total energy needed.

energy expenditure   The amount of energy, measured in calories, that a person uses to breathe, circulate blood, digest food, maintain posture, and be physically active.

ephedrine   A sympathomimetic drug that can be used as an appetite suppressant; it stimulates thermogenesis, or the generation of body heat.

epidemic   The occurrence of more cases of a disease than would be expected in a community or region during a given time period. From the Greek *epi-* (upon) + *demos*, (people or population).

fat   A major source of energy in the diet. All food fats have 9 calories per gram. Fat stores in the body are called adipose tissue.

fenfluramine   A weight-loss drug in a class of drugs called anorectics that decrease appetite. This drug, sold in the United States under the brand name Pondimin, was withdrawn from the U.S. market in 1997 because of its association with heart valve dysfunction.

gastric banding   An obesity surgery option that limits the amount of food the stomach can hold by sectioning it off with a band near its upper end. The band creates a small pouch, which delays the emptying of food from the pouch and causes a feeling of fullness.

gastric bypass   A surgical procedure that combines the creation of a small stomach pouch to restrict food intake with the construction of a bypass of the duodenum to prevent food absorption of some food.

genotype   Describes the entire genetic makeup of an individual or the hereditary factors that define the fundamental constitution of an organism.

glucose   A building block for most carbohydrates. Digestion causes some carbohydrates to break down into glucose. After digestion, glucose is carried in the blood and goes to body cells, where it is used for energy or is stored.

high blood pressure   Hypertension. An optimal blood pressure is less than 120/80 mmHg. With high blood pressure, the heart works harder and chances of a stroke, heart attack, and kidney problems are greater.

hypertension   Abnormally elevated blood pressure.

incidence   The rate at which a certain event occurs. In epidemiology, it is the number of new cases of a specific disease occurring during a certain period.

insulin   A hormone made by the pancreas that helps move glucose (sugar) from the blood to muscles and other tissues. Insulin controls blood sugar levels.

Kcal   Kilocalorie.

LBM   Lean body mass; the weight of the body minus the fat mass.

LCD   Low-calorie diet; a caloric restriction of about 800 to 1,500 calories (approximately 12 to 15 kcal/kg of body weight) per day.

leptin   A hormone secreted by fat cells that has a central role in fat metabolism. Leptin was originally thought to be a signal to lose weight, but it may instead be a signal to the brain that there is fat in the body.

Lipase   An enzyme found in the bowel that assists in lipid absorption by the body.

lipids   Organic (carbon containing) substances that do not dissolve in water. Lipids include fats, waxes, and related compounds.

macronutrients   Nutrients in the diet that are the key sources of energy, namely protein, fat, and carbohydrates.

meta-analysis   Process of using statistical methods to combine the results of different studies. A frequent application is pooling the results from a set of randomized controlled trials, none of which alone is powerful enough to demonstrate statistical significance.

metabolic   Relating to metabolism, the whole range of biochemical processes that occur within living organisms. Metabolism consists of anabolism (the buildup of substances) and catabolism (the breakdown of substances). The term is commonly used to refer specifically to the breakdown of food and its transformation into energy.

metabolic syndrome   A disorder characterized by a cluster of health problems including increased waist circumference, high blood pressure, and abnormal lipid and blood sugar levels.

normal weight   A classification of BMI between 18.5 and 24.9.

nutrition   The process of the body using food to sustain life; the study of food and diet.

obesity   An excessive amount of body fat in relation to lean body mass, or a body weight. It is a BMI of 30 or greater.

obesogenic   Environmental factors that may promote obesity and encourage the expression of a genetic predisposition to gain weight.

orlistat   A lipase inhibitor used for weight loss by reducing the amount of fat the body absorbs by about 30 percent.

OTC   Over the counter; refers to nonprescription drugs.

overweight   An excess of body weight but not necessarily body fat; a body mass index of 25 to 29.9.

pharmacotherapy   Treatment of disease through the use of drugs.

phentermine   A drug used as an anorectic.

prevalence   The total number of cases of a disease in a given population at a specific time.

protein   One of the three nutrients that provide calories to the body. Protein is an essential nutrient that helps build many parts of the body, including muscle, bone, skin, and blood. Protein provides 4 calories per gram and is found in foods like meat, fish, poultry, eggs, dairy products, beans, nuts, and tofu.

RCT   Randomized controlled trial; an experiment in which subjects are randomly allocated into groups to receive or not receive an experimental prevention or therapeutic product. RCTs are generally regarded as the most scientifically rigorous method of hypothesis testing available.

RMR   Resting metabolic rate; accounts for 65 to 75 percent of daily energy expenditure and represents the minimum energy needed to maintain all physiological cell functions in the resting state. The principal determinant of RMR is lean body mass.

satiation   Feeling of fullness that controls the meal size and duration.

satiety   Quality or state of being fed or gratified to or beyond capacity.

sedentary   Having low activity or exercise levels.

sibutramine   A drug used for management of obesity that helps reduce food intake.

SSRI   Selective serotonin reuptake inhibitor; a neurochemical that enhances satisfaction from eating.

systolic blood pressure   The maximum pressure in the artery produced as the heart contracts and blood begins to flow.

type 2 diabetes   The most common form of diabetes; occurs when the body is resistant to the action of insulin and the pancreas cannot make sufficient insulin to overcome this resistance; can be associated with obesity.

underwater weighing   A method for determining body composition; also called hydrostatic weighing.

VLCD   Very-low-calorie diet; a doctor-supervised diet that typically uses commercially prepared formulas to promote rapid weight loss in patients who are moderately to extremely obese. People on a VLCD consume about 800 calories per day or less.

Index